The Nature of Multiple Sclerosis

Papers by
Paavo Riekkinen, Roy L. Swank, John
F. Simpson, John F. Kurtzke, Geoffrey
Dean, Mariella Fischer-Williams,
Hans Link, E. A. Caspary, Oldrich J.
Kolar, Bengt Kallen, Helge Hedberg,
E. J. Field et al.

MSS Information Corporation
655 Madison Avenue, New York, N.Y. 10021

Library of Congress Cataloging in Publication Data
Main entry under title:

The Nature of multiple sclerosis.

    CONTENTS: Riekkinen [and others] Studies on the
pathogenesis of multiple sclerosis: basic proteins in
the myelin and white matter of multiple sclerosis,
subacute sclerosing panencephalitis and postvaccinal
leucoencephalitis. [etc.]
    1. Multiple sclerosis. I. Riekkinen, Paavo.
[DNLM: 1. Multiple sclerosis--Collected works.
WL 360 N285 1973]
RC377.N38 1972   616.8'34'008   72-13055
ISBN 0-8422-7070-1

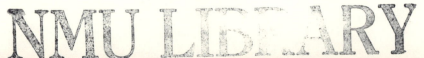

TABLE OF CONTENTS

CREDITS AND ACKNOWLEDGMENTS

Caspary, E. A.; and M. E. Chambers, "Antibody to Encephalitogenic Basic Protein in Multiple Sclerosis and other Neurological Diseases as Measured by Immune Adherence," *European Neurology*, 1970, 3:206-210.

Caspary, E. A.; and E. J. Field, "Sensitization of Blood Lymphocytes to Possible Antigens in Neurological Disease," *European Neurology*, 1970, 4:257-266.

Dean, Geoffrey, "Multiple Sclerosis in Migrants to South Africa," *Israel Journal of Medical Sciences*, 1971, 7:1568.

Field, E. J.: and E. A. Caspary, "Lymphocyte Response Depressive Factor in Multiple Sclerosis," *British Medical Journal*, 1971, 4:529-532.

Fischer-Williams, Mariella; and Ronald C. Roberts, "Cerebrospinal Fluid Proteins and Serum Immunoglobulins: Occurrence in Multiple Sclerosis and Other Neurological Diseases: Comparative Measurement of y-Globulin and the IgG Class," *Archives of Neurology*, 1971, 25:526-534.

Hedberg, Helge; B. Kallen; B. Low; and O. Nilsson, "Impaired Mixed Leucocyte Reaction in Some Different Diseases, Notably Multiple Sclerosis and Various Arthritides," *Clinical and Experimental Immunology*, 1971, 9:201-217.

Kallen, Bengt; and Olle Nilsson, "Mixed Leucocyte Reaction in Multiple Sclerosis," *Nature*, 1971, 22:91-92.

Kolar, Oldrich J.; Alexander T. Ross; and Jean T. Herman, "Serum and Cerebrospinal Fluid Immunoglobulins in Multiple Sclerosis," *Neurology*, 1970, 20:1052-1061.

Kurtzke, J. F., "Some Epidemiologic Features Compatible with an Infectious Origin for Multiple Sclerosis," *International Archives of Allergy*, 1969, 36:59-81.

Kurtzke, John F.; Gilbert W. Beebe, Benedict Nagler, M. Dean Nefzger; Thomas L. Auth; and Leonard T. Kurland, "Studies on the Natural History of Multiple Sclerosis," *Archives of Neurology*, 1970, 22:215-225.

Kurtzke, John F.; Leonard T. Kurland; and Irving D. Goldberg, "Mortality and Migration in Multiple Sclerosis," *Neurology*, 1971, 21:1186-1197.

Link, Hans; and Ragnar Muller, "Immunoglobulins in Multiple Sclerosis and Infections of the Nervous System," *Archives of Neurology*, 1971, 25:326-344.

Riekkinen, P.J.; J. Clausen; H. J. Frey; T. Fog; and U. K. Rinne, "Acid Proteinase Activity of White Matter and Plaques in Multiple Sclerosis," *Acta Neurologica Scandinavia*, 1970, 46:349-353.

Riekkinen, P. J.; Jorma Palo; Antti U. Arstila; Heikki J. Savolainen; Urpo K. Rinne; Erkki K. Kivalo; and Harry Frey, "Protein Composition of Multiple Sclerosis Myelin," *Archives of Neurology*, 1971, 24:545-49.

Riekkinen, P. J.; U. K. Rinne; A. U. Arstila; T. Kurihara; and T. T. Pelliniemi, "Studies on the Pathogenesis of Multiple Sclerosis: 2', 3'-Cyclic Nucleotide 3-Phosphohydrolase as Marker of Demyelination and Correlation of Findings with Lysosomal Changes," *Journal of the Neurological Sciences*, 1972, 15:113-120.

Riekkinen, P. J.; U. K. Rinne; H. Savolainen; J. Palo; E. Kivalo; and A. Arstila, "Studies on the Pathogenesis of Multiple Sclerosis: Basic Proteins in the Myelin and White Matter of Multiple Sclerosis, Subacute Sclerosing Panencephalitis and Postvaccinal Leucoencephalitis," *European Neurology*, 1971, 5:229-244.

Simpson, John F.; Wallace W. Tourtellotte; Empre Kokmen; Julius A. Parker; and Hideo H. Itabashi, "Flourescent Protein Tracing in Multiple Sclerosis Brain Tissue," *Archives of Neurology*, 1969, 20:373-377.

Swank, Roy L., "Multiple Sclerosis: Twenty Years on Low Fat Diet," Archives of Neurology, 1970, 23:460-474.

PREFACE

A chronic neurological disease, multiple sclerosis (M.S.) affects from 10 to 60 people per 100,000 population in the United States alone. Yet the etiology of M.S. is still unknown. We do know that its incidence varies according to graphical latitude and that its early course is characterized by relapses and remissions. The average duration may exceed 25 years as the patient progresses to a bed-ridden, paralyzed, incoordinate, incontinent dysarthric state before death.

Present evidence suggests the involvement of an infectious agent as well as the immune mechanism. The infectious agent is probably viral, for it has been observed that M.S. patients exposed to such other viruses as measles and mumps often have higher measles or mumps antibody titers than titers in controls. Some M.S. patients have high immunoglobulin levels in the cerebrospinal fluid which also suggests that an infectious agent is associated with the disease. Inclusion bodies and small multi-nucleated giant cells have been found in demyelinating scarred areas of the brain from M.S. patients, thus further implicating viruses.

Immunological processes also play a part in the genesis of M.S. Patients often have cellular responses to nervous tissue antigens, lymphotoxic as well as lymphocyte response depressive factors in their serum, and demonstrate impaired mixed leucocyte reactions. However, at this juncture one cannot determine if M.S. is an autoimmune disease or if the immune mechanism is involved as a consequence of a viral infection. It is clear that the course of the disease is highly complex, thereby taxing the clinician in terms of treatment and prognosis.

This volume surveys the recent developments in the areas of pathology, epidemiology, virology, and immunology. It will serve as a reference tool for both beginners and experienced investigators wishing to update their knowledge on this serious and problematic disease.

Ronald Acton, Ph.D.
November, 1972

Pathogenesis of the Disease

Studies on the Pathogenesis of Multiple Sclerosis

Basic Proteins in the Myelin and White Matter of Multiple Sclerosis,
Subacute Sclerosing Panencephalitis and Postvaccinal Leucoencephalitis

P. Riekkinen, U. K. Rinne, H. Savolainen, J. Palo,
E. Kivalo and A. Arstila

During recent years there have been 2 main approaches in studies concerning the etiology and pathogenesis of multiple sclerosis (MS). Both of them, slow virus infection and neuroallergy were reviewed recently from a clinical standpoint by Bauer [1970]. World wide epidemiological data and virological studies suggest an early childhood infection as the origin of the disease [Alter, 1968; Sever et al., 1970; Kurtzke, 1970]. Furthermore, there are reports about specific involvement with measles in MS [Mai, 1969; Adams et al., 1970; Panelius et al., 1970]. The role of environmental factors were also stressed by

KURTZKE [1969] and LEIBOWITZ [1971]. Despite this progress there is still no evidence that slow virus infection explains the whole pathogenesis of MS. Although in subacute sclerosing panencephalitis (SSPE) the association of measles is firmly established [HORTA-BARBOSA *et al.*, 1969] there remain many problems concerning the development of the disease.

The second approach in the search for the pathogenesis has been experimental allergic encephalomyelitis (EAE). Both immunochemical and morphological studies have provided important results as far as oligodendroglia cells and myelin are concerned as targets of immunological attact. Earlier many differences were stressed between lesions of MS and EAE. From the clinical standpoint the most difficult task has been the explanation of the monophasic course of EAE [LAMPERT, 1967; RAINE *et al.*, 1969; BORNSTEIN, 1968; ADAMS and LIEBOVITZ, 1969; LEVINE, 1970]. Although a chronic course for EAE was claimed by STONE and LERNER [1965] only the most recent studies by RAINE and BORNSTEIN [1970] have demonstrated clearly the fact that long-term treatment of tissue cultures with EAE serum causes changes typical of sclerotic plaques. Moreover they demonstrated changes in synaptic membranes before demyelination was apparent.

The main reason for immunochemical studies has been the unique nature of myelin because it contains basic protein which is also called encephalitogen. This protein has been characterised in detail [EINSTEIN and CHAO, 1970; CHAO and EINSTEIN, 1970; ADAMS and CASPARY, 1970; MEHL and HALARIS, 1970; WESTALL *et al.*, 1971; CARNEGIE, 1971]. Antibodies to encephalitogenic protein have also been much studied especially in sera of MS patients, but the results are conflicting [LISAK *et al.*, 1968; CASPARY and CHAMBERS, 1970; LUMSDEN and JENNINGS, 1970]. It has been proposed that demyelinating antibodies are merely a response to demyelination and have little to do with the origin of a demyelination process. However, it has been demonstrated recently by numerous authors [HALLPIKE *et al.*, 1970; EINSTEIN *et al.*, 1970; RIEKKINEN *et al.*, 1971] that basic protein was lost in MS plaques and decreased in many areas outside them. This finding may simply be related to early myelin breakdown because the basic protein is susceptible to proteolysis.

The encephalitogenic protein is not normally exposed to immunocompetent cells and its liberation can cause 2 immunological responses, namely the production of myelin antibodies or the transformation of lymphocytes which can later attack myelin and cause demyelination. This point of view has been expressed [BARTFELD and ATOYNATAN, 1970; DAU and PETERSON, 1970]. However, the specificity of this reaction was questioned by FIELD and CASPARY [1970].

Our previous studies have shown that basic protein decreased in MS myelin samples [RIEKKINEN et al., 1971a] and in SSPE myelin [RIEKKINEN et al., 1971b] our study showed normal content of basic protein. In order to exclude the possibility that the loss of basic protein was due to preparative artefacts during successive gradient centrifugation we went on to study homogenates. In the present study we report the results of further study of MS myelin samples and special emphasis will be paid to the analysis of proteolipids and basic protein in MS white matter homogenates. A comparison is made between MS, SSPE and postvaccinal leucoencephalitis, because it has been suggested that the latter condition is based on immunological responses.

Material and Methods

MS patients

Case 1: A 65-year-old woman, who had suffered from multiple sclerosis for 17 years. The diagnosis was based both on clinical follow-up and on CSF findings. The patient died of respiratory infection and at autopsy several plaques and microscopic features typical of MS were found. The sample for the present study was taken from the temporal area.

Case 2: A 38-year-old man who had had the disease actively for 9 years with typical course and pathology in CSF γ-globulins. The clinical picture was dominated mainly by paraparesis and profuse cerebellar symptoms. At autopsy macroscopic dilatation of ventricles was found and extensive demyelination in many areas. Also in this case the sample was taken from the left temporal white matter.

Case 3: A 47-year-old man, who had had multiple sclerosis for 20 years. The diagnosis was based both on the clinical course and repeated CSF findings. The patient died of a heart attack. At autopsy numerous small periventricular plaques were found and histopathological findings confirmed the diagnosis. The sample for chemical analysis was taken from the left temporo-occipital area outside visible plaque.

Case 4: A 39-year-old woman, in whom the disease had startet at the age of 19 years. Her condition declined continuously and typical CSF for MS was found. At autopsy it was confirmed that the patient had been suffering from multiple sclerosis.

Case 5: A 38-year-old woman who had had the disease for 15 years and had had numerous active attacks and a gradual progression of the disease. Both the clinical picture and CFS findings were in accord with multiple sclerosis. At autopsy plaques were found. Histopathological examination showed typical changes for MS. For the present study a sample was taken from the left anterior temporal area outside the visible plaque.

Cases 6 and 7: (Aged 46 and 58 years) were diagnosed as MS both on the basis of clinical and histopathological findings. Samples were sent from MS tissue Bank Ann Arbor, Mich., USA.

Case 8: A 48-year-old man, whose disease was diagnosed at the age of 31 years. Both clinical data and CSF findings were strongly suggestive of MS. He died of ulcus perforation. Autopsy was performed within 4 h. At autopsy one great plaque was found in the pons and numerous smaller plaques in the periventricular areas. Histopathological finding was typical for MS. For light microscopic control and chemical studies samples were taken from the temporal area outside plaques.

SSPE patients

Case 1: An 18-year-old man with a very acute course of the disease and a typical clinical picture of SSPE including also EEG and CSF data. The patient died 6 months after discovery of the symptoms and autopsy confirmed the diagnosis. White matter was taken from the right temporal lobe.

Case 2: A 15-year-old girl who had had the disease for 2 years, all features clearly pointing to subacute sclerosing panencephalitis including typical CSF. At autopsy atrophy both in white and gray matter was found, especially in occipital areas. Histopathological examination showed extensive demyelination. For the present study left occipital white matter was used.

Postvaccinal leucoencephalitis: A 17-year-old girl, who had been hospitalised in childhood, on accound of allergic manifestation was vaccinated against smallpox. After a week she got a temperature and was treated with tetracycline. On the following day she complained of stiffness in the neck and headache. She had an epileptic seizure and lost consciousness in hospital later the same day. The patient was transferred to the Department of Neurology, University of Turku, and when admitted to the department she was unconscious and was placed immediately in an artificial respirator. CSF contained 12 white cells/mm^3 and IgG content of CSF was 33% of total proteins. She died after 24 h and at autopsy numerous haemorrhagic areas were found, mainly in white matter and also foreign cell infiltrates around veins were seen.

Control samples were taken at autopsies from cases who had no clinical symptoms suggestive of MS or a related disease. Both the site of samples and the time period after death corresponded with those of MS cases. The average age of the control patients was 57 years and 7 were male and 3 female.

Dissection of samples and light microscopic control: From every sample of white matter a part was taken for light microscopic study and the rest was used for chemical analyses and separation of myelin. For light microscopic examination the samples were embedded in paraffin and myelin sheaths were stained with Luxol Fast Blue, MBS.

Separation of myelin: This was according to the method presented in an earlier connection by RUMSBY et al. [1970]. Briefly it consists of homogenization of white matter in 0.32 M sucrose at the pH 7.35. After homogenization cell debris and crude particles are removed by pelletting 3 times at 1,000 g for 5 min. After every sedimentation only the supernatant is taken. The final supernatant was spun down 3 times at 13,500 g for 10 min in order to get the crude mitochondrial fraction. The supernatant from these runs was discarded each time and the sediment re-homogenized in the original volume of 0.32 M sucrose. The crude fraction which contained myelin, mitochondria and other membrane material was fractionated further in the discontinous sucrose gradient against 0.656 M sucrose (40,000 g and running time 30 min). After the run the white myelin layer was recovered from the interphase and diluted with water so that the final sucrose concentration was 0.32 M. After 2 runs osmotic shock treatment was carried out and then 3rd gradient centrifugation was performed. Finally, a 2nd osmotic shock treatment was carried out and then the myelin was spun down as white pellet at 13,500 g for 10 min.

Biochemiacl evaluation of myelin contamination: The purity of the final myelin preparations was evaluated for every sample by using acid phosphatase as a marker for lysosomal contamination, as described by RIEKKINEN and CLAUSEN [1969] and SDH as a marker for mitochondrial contamination [RUMSBY et al., 1970]. Protein (from dry weight) was analysed, using Lowry's method [LOWRY et al., 1951].

Electron microscopy: For quantitative morphometric analysis of myelin the samples were fixed in a suspension of 0.1 M Na-cacodylate buffer with 3% glutaraldehyde for 3 h, washed and postfixed with 1% Na-cacodylate, buffered (OsO$_4$) with osmium tetroxide, for 1 h. The samples were then collected on Millipore filters and prepared for morphometry as described by FREY et al. [1970]. Both intact and broken myelin lamellae were analysed and also contamination.

Electrophoretic protein analysis. This was made according to the method described by MEHL and HALARIS [1970] and EINSTEIN et al. [1970]. Details of the procedure will be found in a previous report [RIEKKINEN et al., 1971]. 15% horizontal polyacrylamide gel was used as carrier medium and phenol-formic acid-water (14:3:3) solvent in plastic tanks. The gels were stained with amido black. Purified basic protein was used as a reference in addition to cytochrome c. Scanning analyses were performed using Canalco Model E microdensitometer.

Results

Myelin recovery: As mentioned in the methods section no visible plaques were found in MS samples, but light microscopic evaluation revealed perivascular cell infiltrates in many samples. When standard procedure was used for separation of myelin it was found that the amount of myelin obtained from MS cases was lower than in control material.

In SSPE cases the bulk of the floating material above the gradient was seen but this was not taken for analysis. The amount of myelin was also in these cases greatly decreased.

14

Protein content: The protein content of myelin samples varied in MS material from 172 to 235 μg/mg dry weight. In control material corresponding values were 210 and 262. For SSPE cases the values were 207 and 279. These values for myelin protein contents are in accordance with those reported by others recently [MURDOCK *et al.*, 1969].

Electron microscopic control of myelin samples: Both qualitative inspections and quantitative morphometric analyses showed mainly well-preserved multilamellar myelin structures and empty axonal space. However, in many samples broken membrane material was found which seemed to originate from intact myelin. We could not identify any microsomes or lysosomes. When some remnants of axonal content were left, mitochondria-like destroyed particles were found.

Biochemical criteria of purity: From every myelin preparation microsomal, mitochondrial and lysosomal enzymes were assayed in order to reveal possible contamination by various cellular structures. When detected values were compared with corresponding data of original homogenate only traces of acid phosphatase and SDH activity were demonstrated in myelin which argued that our myelin samples were suitable for electrophoretic analysis.

Protein composition of MS myelin: We have previously reported that the amount of basic protein was decreased in MS myelin. In agreement with our earlier results are electrophoretic data presented in figure 1, No. 1–5 are control samples and No. 6–11 MS cases. Our data showed clearly that the amount of basic protein was decreased in those samples where the major proteolipid fraction was normal. As can be seen from

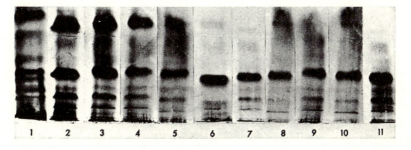

Fig. 1. Electrophoretic patterns of control and MS myelin samples. No. 1–5 are controls. No. 6–10 are from the 5 first-mentioned MS cases (see text) and No. 11 from MS case 8. Far moving band is basic protein. For other details see the text.

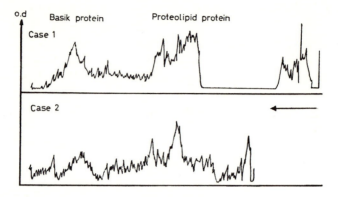

Fig. 2. Scanning curves of 2 purified SSPE myelin samples. The arrow shows the direction of electrophoretic run. Note the normal proportion of basic protein and double band of proteolipid protein in SSPE case 1.

the electropherograms the most important finding was the proportion of various proteins.

Protein composition of SSPE myelin: In figure 2 will be seen typical scanning patterns of 2 SSPE myelin samples purified with the same sub-cellular fractionation method as the myelin samples. The striking difference was the normal proportion of various proteins in the SSPE cases. The basic protein did not show any remarkable decrease when compared with proteolipid proteins. In one of our SSPE samples we also found a double band in the major proteolipid fraction in successive runs. However, the other SSPE myelin showed the usual proteolipid pattern. The results confirmed our earlier findings.

Protein composition of white matter homogenate in MS, SSPE and postvaccinal leucoencephalitis with special reference to basic protein: Freeze-dried material originally-homogenized 100 mg/ml in water was dissolved in the same way as the myelin [EINSTEIN *et al.,* 1970] in phenol, acetic acid and water. Some basic proteins like histones and ribosomal basic proteins move towards the cathode but not exactly in the same position as the myelin basic protein and their amount is also lower and they do not disturb the electrophoreses as strikingly as the lipids. It seemed that in homogenate material the free or membrane-bound lipids were the most serious source of error. Some proteins also stuck at the

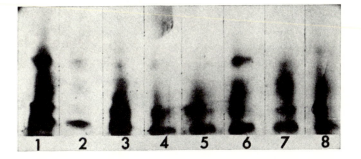

Fig. 3. Electrophoretic distribution of proteolipid proteins and basic protein in freeze-dried white matter homogenate. No. 1 and 6 are controls. No. 2–5 are from the 4 first-mentioned MS cases. No. 7 and 8 are from SSPE cases 1 and 2, respectively. Note the decrease of basic protein (far moving band in controls) in MS and SSPE cases.

starting point and thus caused a disturbance in the normal mobility of different membrane proteins.

It can be seen in the figure 3 (No. 2–5), that the amount of basic protein was decreased in MS homogenates when compared with controls.

In figure 4 are the scanning patterns of some MS samples and in figure 5 those of controls. It can be seen that when compared with controls the proportion of basic protein was decreased in MS. In figure 3 (No. 7 and 8) are results for SSPE white matter samples. They show that also in SSPE white matter basic protein was decreased in contrast to findings in myelin (fig. 2). Although only one postvaccinal leucoencephalitis case has as yet been analysed by us figure 6 shows a pronounced decrease of basic protein in this sample. In this case a profuse demyelination was found on the basis of myelin staining and lipid data.

Discussion

A comment on the different methods: It was possible to identify the absence of plaques and also in some cases to observe a diffuse infiltration of mononuclear cells and thin myelin sheaths. In agreement with this were our results concerning myelin recovery which was constantly lower in MS and SSPE samples.

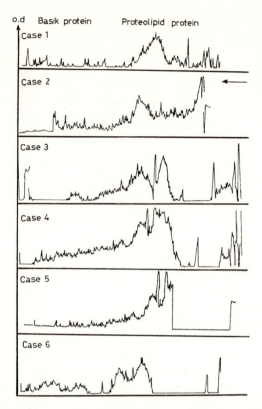

Fig. 4. Scanning curves of the 6 first-mentioned MS cases. In all cases freeze-dried homogenate material was run and the proportion of major proteolipid protein and basic protein was scanned. Note the marked decrease of basic protein area.

In all studies where samples are from autopsy material one must be careful in interpreting the results obtained. However, there seems to be little variation in the chemical composition reported by different authors [MOKRASCH, 1969] for human CNS myelin purified from white matter. Our separation method has shown clearly reproducible results [RUMSBY et al., 1970; FREY et al., 1970].

In all electrophoretic runs MS and other pathological samples were analysed together with controls. Although freezing and thawing can cause differences in our study both fresh and frozen samples gave identi-

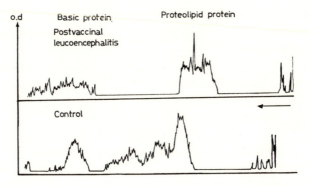

Fig. 5. Representative scanning curves for control white matter homogenate showing the normal proportions of proteolipid protein and basic protein.

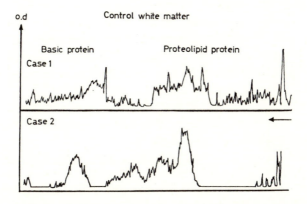

Fig. 6. Scanning patterns of postvaccinal leucoencephalitis and control white matter homogenate. Note the decrease of basic protein in the postvaccinal leucoencephalitis case.

cal results. Our results for myelin were more constant. In total homogenate material lipids and proteins originating from other fractions contributed significantly to the fact that proteins stuck at the starting point.

Interpretation of the results and their significance in demyelination: The basic protein or encephalitogenic fragment of the myelin sheath has been an object of intensive research mainly from the immunochemical standpoint. It was demonstrated by ENG *et al.* [1968] that the basic protein of myelin is also very characteristic for adult myelin. In later de-

19

tailed studies it was shown that encephalitogen grandually appears in myelin [EINSTEIN *et al.*, 1970]. On the basis of these results it seems to be essential for the structural maintainance of the myelin sheath. Both in the peripheral nerve and in CNS myelin this protein is lost in an early step of demyelination [HALLPIKE *et al.*, 1970] because the basic protein is a vulnerable part and especially liberated by proteolytic enzymes from the myelin sheath [HALLPIKE and ADAMS, 1969].

The main question is whether encephalitogenic protein and its liberation can contribute to the pathogenesis of multiple sclerosis. There have been conflicting opinions about antibodies to basic protein in multiple sclerosis [CASPARY and CHAMBERS, 1970; LUMSDEN and JENNINGS, 1970] and the problem is more complicated where *in vitro* demyelinating antibodies and their occurrence is concerned [DOWLING *et al.*, 1969; KIM *et al.*, 1970] because the presence of such antibodies has been demonstrated both in serum and CSF. However, the findings are not specific for multiple sclerosis. If encephalitogenic protein is liberated its presence in serum and CSF should be demonstrable and in fact this has been done for CSF [MCPHERSON *et al.*, 1970]. Furthermore, in serum it seems that the α-globulin fraction can bind encephalitogenic protein [MCPHERSON *et al.*, 1970].

An attempt has been made to determine the role of lymphocytes using purified lymphocyte fractions and their sensitization by different antigens. HUGUES *et al.* [1968] came to the conclusion that lymphocyte transformation did not differ significantly in MS material towards encephalitogenic protein when compared with other neurological patients. On the other hand in some later studies where both well-purified encephalitogenic protein and lymphocyte fractions were used a difference was found in the responses of lymphocytes between MS and other neurological patients [DAU and PETERSON, 1970; BARTFELD and ATOYNATAN, 1970]. These results suggest some role for lymphocytes in the early pathogenesis of the disease because in brain biopsy material plasma cells or lymphocytes have also been found [SLUGA, 1969] and our own electron microscopic observations have in some cases shown lymphocytes also in white matter biopsy specimens.

Although serological studies strongly suggest a measles virus infection as a cause of MS it may be that demyelinating antibodies and cell mediated immunocyte responses are involved in the pathogenesis of multiple sclerosis; this has been shown for Guillain-Barré syndrome by COOK *et al.* [1970, 1971]. Our present results show differences in the mechanism of demyelination when these different diseases are compared. In SSPE all the myelin lamellae are digested without selective involvement of protein constituents but in MS the myelin is not degraded *in toto* but the basic protein may be lost in an early step before the proteolipids. It remains to be seen whether reactive changes of glia or inflammatory cells are a primary cause of these early changes in the disease. There is final proof that in MS and related diseases the pathological immuno-globulins appearing in CSF are produced in CSN [TOURTELLOTTE, 1970] but the antigens of these antibodies are completely unknown. There is no evidence that these pathological immunoglobulins are specific to some antigenic determinants but at least in SSPE, measles antibodies are located in this fraction.

It is difficult to say whether both glia and myelin are targets for im-munocytolysis but as far as encephalitogenic protein is concerned, at the present time the bulk of the evidence shows that it is present only in the myelin sheath and so the antibodies or demyelinating factors described by BORNSTEIN [1968] as attacking both myelin and oligodendroglia cells are not just antibodies towards basic protein.

DICKINDSON *et al.* [1970] have put forward the hypothesis that encepha-litogenic protein is lost from the myelin sheath spontaneously with-out the involvement of enzymatic reactions and the same authors have questioned the evidence that proteolysis is the basic cause of this pheno-men [WHOLMAN, 1965; PORCELLATI, 1970; HALLPIKE *et al.,* 1970; RIEK-KINEN *et al.,* 1970]. Therefore, it still remains to be proved that the in-creased proteolysis in active areas of demyelination and decrease of bas-ic proteins will have immunological consequences.

The concept of neuroallergy has been stressed in many connections [POSER, 1969] and its significance for the development of postinfectious and postvaccinal encephalitis and encephalomyelitis is broadly docu-mented on the basis of the antigenic properties of myelin. Our present data for postinfectious leucoencephalitis show that during the disease process encephalitogenic protein is lost from white matter but not selec-tively from myelin. The significance of myelin antigenic properties in the development of different demyelinating diseases remains to be proved.

It is difficult to understand the appearance of the clinical symptoms of acute MS only on the basis of demyelination. It is more probable that inflammatory factors play a major role and a functional block in the synapses for neuronal transmission due to immunocytolysis has been suggested [CARNEGIE, 1971]. Moreover, it seems that basic protein also exists in the synaptosomal membrane [FISZER and DEROBERTIS, 1969]. This may open up a new aspect concerning the appearance of clinical signs.

Acknowledgements

We wish to thank Miss K. LINDBERG and Miss L. TÖRMÄNEN for technical assistance. This study was supported by grant from The National Research Council for Medical Sciences, Finland.

References

ADAMS, C. W. M. and LEIBOWITZ, S.: The general pathology of demyelinating diseases; in BOURNE The structure and function of nervous tissue. Biochemistry and disease, vol. 3, p. 309 (Academic Press, New York 1969).

ADAMS, R. D. and CASPARY, E. A.: The relationship between encephalitogenic factor and myelin. J. neurol. Sci. *11:* 187 (1970).

ADAMS, J. M.; BROOKS, M.; FISHER, E. D., and TYLER, C. S.: Measles antibodies in patients with multiple sclerosis and with other neurological and nonneurological diseases. Neurology, Minneap. *20:* 1039 (1970).

ALTER, M.: Etiological considerations based on the epidemiology of multiple sclerosis. Amer. J. Epidem. *88:* 318 (1968).

BARTFELD, H. and ATOYNATAN, T.: Lymphocyte transformation in multiple sclerosis. Brit. med. J. *ii:* 91 (1970).

BAUER, H. J.: Multiple Sklerose. Grundlagen und Hypothesen der modernen Ursachenforschung. J. Neurol. *198:* 5 (1970).

BORNSTEIN, M. B.: Central nervous system. Textbook of immunopathology, vol. 2, p. 507 (Grune & Stratton, New York 1968).

CARNEGIE, P. R.: Properties, structure and possible neuroreceptor role of the encephalitogenic protein of human brain. Nature, Lond. *229:* 25 (1971).

CASPARY, E. A. and CHAMBERS, M. E.: Antibody to encephalitogenic basic protein in multiple sclerosis and other neurological diseases as measured by immune adherence. Europ. Neurol. *3:* 206 (1970).

CHAO, L.-P. and EINSTEIN, E. R.: Localization of the active site through chemical modification of the encephalitogenic protein. J. biol. Chem. *245:* 6397 (1970).

COOK, S. T.; DOWLING, P. C., and WHITAKER, J. N.: The Guillain-Barre syndrome. Relationship of circulating immunocytes to desease activity. Arch. Neurol., Chicago *22:* 470 (1970).

COOK, S. T.; DOWLING, P. C.; MURRAY, M. R., and WHITAKER, J. N.: Circulating demyelinating factors in acute idiopathic polyneuropathy. Arch. Neurol., Chicago *24:* 136 (1971).

DAU, P. C. and PETERSON, R. D. A.: Transformation of lymphocytes from patients with multiple sclerosis. Use of an encephalitogenic of human origin, with a report of a trial of immunosuppressive therapy in multiple sclerosis. Arch. Neurol., Chicago *23:* 32 (1970).

DICKINSON, J. P.; JONES, K. M.; APARICIO, S. R., and LUMSDEN, C. E.: Localization of encephalitogenic basic protein in the intraperiodic line of lamellar myelin. Nature, Lond. *227:* 1133 (1970).

DOWLING, P. C.; KIM, S. U.; MURRAY, M. R., and COOK, S. T.: Serum 19 S and 7 S demyelinating antibodies in multiple sclerosis. J. Immunol. *101:* 1101 (1969).

EINSTEIN, E. R. and CHAO, L.-P.: Problems realted to the protein-eliciting experimental allergic encephalomyelitis. Protein metabolism of the nervous system, p. 643 (Plenum Publishing, New York 1970).

EINSTEIN, E. R.; DALAL, K. B., and CSEJTEY, J.: Increased protease activity and changes in basic proteins and lipids in multiple sclerosis plaques. J. neurol. Sci. *11:* 109 (1970a).

EINSTEIN, E. R.; DALAL, K. B., and CSEJTEY, J.: Biochemical maturation of the central nervous system. 2. Proteins and proteolytic enzyme changes. Brain Res. *18:* 35 (1970b).

ENG, L. F.; CHAO, F.-C.; GERSTL, B.; PRATT, D., and TAVASTJERNA, M. G.: The maturation of human white matter myelin. Fractionation of the myelin membrane proteins. Biochemistry *7:* 4455 (1968).

FIELD, E. J. and CASPARY, E. A.: Lymphocyte sensitisation. An *in vitro* test for cancer. Lancet *ii:* 1337 (1970).

FISZER, S. and DEROBERTIS, E.: Subcellular distribution and chemical nature of the recepter for 5-hydroxytryptamine in the central nervous system. J. Neurochem. *16:* 1201 (1969).

FREY, H. J.; RIEKKINEN, P. J.; RINNE, U. K., and ARSTILA, A. U.: Peptidase activity of myelining the myelination period in guinea-pig brain. Brain Res. *22:* 243 (1970).

HALLPIKE, J. F. and ADAMS, C. W. M.: Proteolysis and myelin breakdown. A review of recent histochemical and biochemical studies. Histochem. J. *1:* 559 (1969).

HALLPIKE, J. F.; ADAMS, C. W. M., and BAYLISS, O. B.: Histochemistry of myelin. XI. Loss of basic protein in early myelin breakdown and multiple sclerosis plaques. Histochem. J. *2:* 323 (1970).

HORTA-BARBOSA, L.; FUCCILLO, D. A., and SEVER, L. J.: Subacute sclerosing panencephalitis. Isolation of measles virus from a brain biopsy. Nature, Lond. *221:* 974 (1969).

HUGHES, D.; CASPARY, E. A., and FIELD, E. J.: Lymphocyte transformation induced by encephalitogenic factor in multiple sclerosis and other neurological diseases. Lancet *ii:* 1205 (1968).

KIM, S. U.; MURRAY, M. R.; TOURTELLOTTE, W. W., and PARKER, J.: Demonstration in tissue culture of myelinotoxicity in cerebrospinal fluid and brain extracts from multiple sclerosis patients. J. Neuropath. exp. Neurol. *24:* 421 (1970).

KURTZKE, J. F.: Some epidemiological features compatible with an infectious origin for multiple sclerosis. Pathogenesis and etiology of demyelinating diseases. Int. Arch. Allergy *36:* add., pp. 59–81 (1969).

KURTZKE, J. F.: Multiple sclerosis as a latent infection of the nervous system. Proc. 6th Int. Congr. Neuropath., Paris, p. 952 (1970).

LAMPERT, P.: Electron microscopic studies on ordinary and hyperacute experimental allergic encephalomyelitis. Acta neuropath. *9:* 99 (1967).

LISAK, R. P.; HEINZE, R. G.; FALK, G. A., and KIES, M. W.: Search for anti-encephalitogen antibody in human demyelinative diseases. Neurology, Minneap. *18:* 122 (1968).

LEIBOWITZ, U.: Multiple sclerosis progress in epidemiological and experimental research. J. neurol. Sci. *12:* 307 (1971).

LEVINE, S.: Allergic encephalomyelitis. Cellular transformation and vascular blockade. J. Neuropath. exp. Neurol. *24:* 6 (1970).

LOWRY, O. H.; ROSEBROUGH, H. J.; FARR, A. L., and RANDALL, R. J.: Protein measurement with the Folin phenol reagent. J. biol. Chem. *193:* 265 (1951).

LUMSDEN, C. E. and JENNINGS, M.: Antimyelin antibodies in multiple sclerosis. Significance for pathogenesis. Proc. 6th Iit. Congr. Neuropath., Paris, p. 489 (1970).

MAI, K.: Measles antibodies in multiple sclerosis patients and controls (biostatistical evaluaton). Pathogenesis and etiology of demyelinating diseases. Int. Arch. Allergy *36:* add., p. 109 (1969).

MCPHERSON, T. A.; ROBSON, G. S. M., and CARNEGIE, P. R.: Is encephalitogenic basic protein in human cerebrospinal fluid? Int. Arch. Allergy *39:* 566 (1970a).

MCPHERSON, T. A.; MARCHALONIS, J. J., and LENNON, V.: Binding of encephalitogenic basic protein by serum α-globulin. Immunology, Lond. *19:* 929 (1970b).

MEHL, E. and HALARIS, A.: Stoichiometric relation of protein components in cerebral myelin from different species. J. Neurochem. *17:* 659 (1970).

MOKRASCH, L. C.: Myelin; in LAJTHA Handbook of neurochemistry, vol. 1, p. 171 (Plenium Publishing, New York 1969).

MURDOCK, D. D.; KATONA, E., and MOSCARELLO, M. A.: Preparation of myelin using the L-4 zonal ultracentrifuge. Canad. J. Biochem. *47:* 818 (1969).

PANELIUS, M.; MYLLYLÄ, G.; PENTTINEN, K.; HALONEN, P., and RINNE, U. K.: Platelet aggregation test with measles antigen in multiple sclerosis. Brit. med. J. *ii:* 461 (1970).

PORCELLATI, G.: Studies on proteinase enzymes during Wallarian degeneration; in LAJTHA Protein metabolism of the nervous system, p. 601 (Plenium Publishing, New York 1970).

POSER, C. M.: Disseminated vasculomyelinopathy. A review of the clinical and pathologic reactions of the nervous system in hyperergic diseases. Acta neurol. scand. *45:* suppl. 37, p.   (1969).

RAINE, C. R. and BORNSTEIN, M. B.: Experimental allergic encephalomyelitis. A light and electron microscopic study of demyelination and sclerosis *in vitro*. J. Neuropath. exp. Neurol. *24:* 552 (1970).

RAINE, C. R.; WISNIESKI, H., and PRINEAS, J.: An ultrastructural study of experimental demyelination and remyelination. II. Chronic experimental allergic encephalomyelitis in the peripheral nervous system. Lab. Invest. *21:* 316 (1969).

RIEKKINEN, P. J.; CLAUSEN, J. C.; FREY, H. J.; FOG, T., and RINNE, U. K.: Acid proteinase activity of white matter and plaques in multiple sclerosis. Acta neurol. scand. *46:* 349 (1970).

RIEKKINEN, P. J.; PALO, J.; ARSTILA, A. U.; RINNE, U. K.; SAVOLAINEN, H.; KIVALO,

E., and FREY, H.: Protein composition of multiple sclerosis myelin. Arch. Neurol., Chicago *24:* 545 (1971).

RIEKKINEN, P. J.; PALO, J.; ARSTILA, A. U.; RINNE, U. K.; FREY, H.; SAVOLAINEN, H., and KIVALO, E.: Protein composition of white matter myelin in subacute sclerosing panencephalitis. J. neurol. Sci. (1971b, in press).

RUMSBY, M. G.; RIEKKINEN, P. J., and ARSTILA, A. U.: A critical evaluation of myelin purification. Nonspecific esterase activity associated with central nerve myelin preparations. Brain Res. *24:* 495 (1970).

SEVER, J. L.; KURTZKE, J. F.; ALTER, M.; SCHUMACHER, G. A., and GILKESON, M. R.: Virus antibodies and multiple sclerosis. Proc. 6th Int. Congr. Neuropath., Paris, p. 958 (1970).

SLUGA, E.: Beitrag zur Feinstruktur der Läsionen bei der Multiplen Sklerose des Menschen. Aktuelle Probleme der Multiplen Sklerose. Wien. Z. Nervenheilk., suppl. 2, p. 59 (1969).

STONE, S. H. and LERNER, E. M.: Chronic disseminated allergic encephalomyelitis in guinea pigs. Ann. N. Y. Acad. Sci. *122:* 227 (1965).

TOURTELLOTTE, W. W.: On cerebrospinal fluid immunoglobulin-G (IgG). Quotients in multiple sclerosis and other diseases. A review and a new formula to estimate the amount of IgG synthesized per day by the central nervous system. J. neurol. Sci. *10:* 279 (1970).

WESTALL, F. C.; ROBINSON, A. B.; CACCAM, J.; JACKSON, J., and EYLAR, E. H.: Essential chemical requirements for induction of allergic encephalomyelitis. Nature, Lond. *229:* 22 (1971).

WHOLMAN, M.: *In vitro* breakdown of myelin. Ann. N. Y. Acad. Sci. *122:* 401 (1965).

Studies on the Pathogenesis of Multiple Sclerosis

2',3'-Cyclic Nucleotide 3-Phosphohydrolase as Marker of Demyelination and Correlation of Findings with Lysosomal Changes

P. J. RIEKKINEN, U. K. RINNE, A. U. ARSTILA, T. KURIHARA AND T. T. PELLINIEMI

INTRODUCTION

It was reported recently that 2',3'-cyclic nucleotide 3'-phosphohydrolase is located mainly in the myelin sheath in the central nervous system (CNS) and only trace amounts were to be found in other structures (Kurihara and Tsukada 1967). The same authors have also shown that the appearance of phosphohydrolase in the CNS coincides with the active period of myelination (Kurihara and Tsukada 1968). These results concerning the association of phosphohydrolase and the myelin sheath have been confirmed in later reports by other authors (Banik and Davison 1969; Olafson, Drummond and Lee 1969).

Although phosphohydrolase is not located only in the myelin sheath it seems to offer a suitable marker for studies dealing with dysmyelination or a demyelinating process. Kurihara, Nussbaum and Mandel (1969, 1970) have shown that in brains of mutant mice with deficient myelination the phosphohydrolase activity was three to four times lower than in corresponding controls. It is firmly established that cerebroside is located mainly in myelin and that its amount corresponds to histological demyelination, *e.g.* in multiple sclerosis (MS) (Adams, Ibrahim and Leibowitz 1965), but phosphohydrolase assay is not so complicated as cerebroside analysis. Accepting the fact that phosphohydrolase, cerebroside and cholesterol are mainly located in myelin, in quantitative terms it is of special importance to compare the results for acid proteinase and acid phosphatase with myelin markers.

Since we have shown previously that multiple sclerosis white matter displays lysosomal changes in areas where lipid composition is quite normal (Rinne, Riekkinen and Arstila 1970) it is of practical importance to correlate phosphohydrolase activity

This study was supported by the Sigrid Juselius Foundation. A part of this study was undertaken during the period of a fellowship awarded to Dr. Kurihara by Emil Aaltonen Foundation.

with corresponding cerebroside data, myelin staining and with activities of lysosomal hydrolases. Such a study may further reveal whether structures other than myelin sheaths, *e.g.* glial cells, react first in MS and demyelination is a secondary response. In order to answer this question the present work was undertaken.

MATERIAL AND METHODS

Patient material

MS cases. Seven patients were diagnosed both on the basis of clinical findings and neuropathological examination as having multiple sclerosis. Typical plaques were found. For the present study white matter was taken from the temporal region outside plaques in these 7 cases. Moreover, from an MS autopsy, samples were taken from different brain areas including plaques and areas at different stages of demyelination.

Two patients dying of subacute sclerosing panencephalitis (SSPE) were also included in our material because demyelination is a rather prominent histopathological feature in SSPE. The corresponding temporal area was taken for analysis.

Control samples were taken at autopsies from patients who had no suspicion of MS or related disease from corresponding brain areas.

Light microscopy

Part of the sample taken for analysis was embedded in paraffin and myelin sheaths were stained with Luxol Fast Blue B. Also hematoxylin eosin and Van Gieson staining were performed for routine examination. The typical absence of myelin sheaths was ascertained in plaques and microscopic demyelinated areas were also found in samples which were normal when inspected visually. In samples from temporal areas occasional cell infiltrates were found.

Homogenization

Tissue was homogenized, 100 mg/ml in distilled water. For enzyme analysis homogenates were assayed immediately and were also repeated later.

2′,3′-Cyclic nucleotide 3-phosphohydrolase was assayed according to the method described in detail by Kurihara *et al.* (1970). Acid *p*-nitrophenyl-phosphatase and acid proteinase were analysed in the manner described by Riekkinen and Clausen (1969). Total cerebrosides were analysed according to the method of Hess and Thalheimer (1965).

Total lipid phosphorus was determined according to Bartlett (1959) with the exception that digestion was made according to Svandborg and Svennerholm (1961). Total cholesterol was analysed according to Badzio and Boczon (1966).

Protein determination was made according to the method of Lowry, Rosebrough, Farr and Randall (1951) using bovine serum albumin as standard.

RESULTS

Light microscopic findings

White matter samples taken from the temporal region of 7 MS cases showed no plaques. However, occasional thin myelin sheaths were found. No gliosis was seen in these areas. In 1 MS sample a striking cellular infiltration was seen (MS Case 1, Table 1) and in other cases a few mononuclear cells were found. In all these cases numerous plaques in other areas and changes typical of MS were found. These included some microscopic plaques which also showed diffuse demyelination and cellular infiltrates. Old plaques showed almost a complete absence of histologically demonstrable myelin.

SSPE samples showed clear cellular infiltrates and also demyelinated areas. However in SSPE samples the changes were not confined so strikingly to myelin sheaths and axonal degeneration was also found.

TABLE 1

COMPARISON OF PHOSPHOHYDROLASE ACTIVITY WITH OTHER FINDINGS IN TEMPORAL WHITE MATTER OF MS AND SSPE AUTOPSY SPECIMENS[a]

Cases	Phospho-hydrolase	Cere-broside	Choles-terol	Phospho-lipids	Acid proteinase	Acid phos-phatase
Multiple sclerosis 1	17.8	123	135	285	62.4	55.7
Multiple sclerosis 2	18.7	145	149	267	25.2	34.2
Multiple sclerosis 3	19.0	156	132	293	34.5	29.6
Multiple sclerosis 4	15.2	119	125	258	26.4	38.2
Multiple sclerosis 5	18.6	147	156	296	38.6	30.4
Multiple sclerosis 6	13.8	112	126	269	25.6	32.1
Multiple sclerosis 7	16.8	143	155	279	43.6	29.6
Mean ± SEM	17.1 ± 0.8	131.0 ± 6.3	139.7 ± 5.1	278.1 ± 5.4	36.8 ± 5.1	35.7 ± 3.5
SSPE acute	13.2	89	106	247	75.4	91.0
SSPE chronic	5.2	68	79	242	60.5	38.1
Controls[b]	19.4 ± 2.4 (11)	146.2 ± 3.9 (16)	152.9 ± 2.9 (16)	297 ± 3.6 (16)	19.4 ± 2.6 (52)	17.9 ± 2.7 (52)

[a] Results for phospholipids, cholesterol and cerebroside are expressed as μg/mg dry weight, acid proteinase as μmoles tyrosine liberated/mg protein/hr, acid phosphatase as μmoles p-nitrophenol released/mg protein/min, phosphohydrolase as μmoles substrate hydrolysed/mg protein/20 min.
[b] Mean ± SEM for control specimens.

Comparison of phosphohydrolase in the temporal region with other changes

Table 1 shows results from 7 MS and 2 SSPE samples. The phosphohydrolase activity was clearly lowest in the chronic SSPE case. In that case phosphohydrolase activity was almost two times lower than in corresponding controls. Another SSPE case which had a more acute clinical course and milder demyelination did not differ so much from controls. All MS cases showed values which were fairly constant and were in the same range as corresponding controls with the exception of Cases 4 and 6 where decreased values were found.

When the cerebroside values are compared case by case in controls and MS cases they show the same trend as phosphohydrolase values. Once again the SSPE case which was less active for phosphohydrolase contained less cerebroside expressed as μg/mg dry weight. The second SSPE case, in agreement with phosphohydrolase, contained a higher amount of cerebroside. Also in MS cases phosphohydrolase activities and cerebroside data showed corresponding changes. Especially this can be seen in MS Cases 4 and 6 (Table 1) where cholesterol values were also lower than in controls. These results for phosphohydrolase and cerebroside were in agreement with slight changes obtained in myelin staining.

Total phospholipids and cholesterol did not reveal any new aspects. In the SSPE cases they were definitely lower and also in those MS cases where cerebroside had decreased.

Acid phosphatase and acid proteinase are mainly markers of lysosomes. From the same table it can be seen that acid proteinase activities increased especially markedly in cases where myelin constituents did not reveal clear changes. The difference between acute and more chronic sclerosing panencephalitis cases was not striking. When SSPE cases are compared with MS the results are also interesting. Although demyelination was apparent in some MS cases the acid hydrolase values were more clearly increased in SSPE.

Phosphohydrolase, cerebroside, acid proteinase and myelin staining in different parts of plaques

Table 2 shows results from the pontine plaque, a large active demyelinated area in the spinal cord, a periventricular plaque and the optic nerves. These results clearly demonstrate the fact that phosphohydrolase activity decreases markedly in plaque areas. In the left optic nerve, where demyelination was almost complete on the basis of myelin staining, phosphohydrolase activity decreased 20 times. On the other hand the large pontine plaque which seemed to be an old one still contained a low level of phosphohydrolase activity. In the spinal cord the activity of phosphohydrolase decreased markedly as did also the number of myelin lamellae in myelin staining. It is apparent that in the plaque area the phosphohydrolase activity increased in the direction of normal white matter when samples were taken from different parts of plaques. Thus although there seems to be some regional variation in cerebroside content the values presented in Table 2 show that cerebroside correlated well with phosphohydrolase activities and also with myelin staining.

Acid proteinase activity increased greatly in areas of active demyelination and es-

TABLE 2

CORRELATION OF VARIOUS CHEMICAL FINDINGS IN DIFFERENT AREAS OF DEMYELINATION IN MS AUTOPSY SAMPLES. RESULTS ARE EXPRESSED AS IN TABLE 1

Place of the sample	Phospho-hydrolase	Cerebro-side	Cholesterol	Phospho-lipids	Acid proteinase
Centre of plaque (pons)	2.12	82	89.3	192	14.8
Border of plaque (pons)	7.42	132	144.0	276	52.6
Spinal cord C2	3.19	108	104.0	209	50.0
Periventricular plaque	5.31	32	121.0	239	51.5
Left optic nerve	0.54	—[a]	—[a]	—[a]	12.0
Right optic nerve	2.11	—[a]	—[a]	—[a]	15.6

[a] Not analysed because of small amount of sample.

pecially around plaques. However in the optic nerves, where demyelination and cellular reaction were already at the inactive stage, the acid proteinase activity decreased. It must be stressed that the results for phosphohydrolase and acid proteinase are quite opposite. Acid proteinase activity increased in the active region of demyelination, whereas phosphohydrolase and other myelin markers showed decreased values.

DISCUSSION

The purpose of the present study was to discover whether phosphohydrolase is a suitable indicator of demyelination in human material in demyelinating diseases and how its activity correlates with myelin staining and cerebroside. On the other hand we have compared indicators of myelin with lysosomal changes.

It has been tentatively suggested by numerous authors that all white matter shows changes in MS, even outside plaques (Cumings 1955; Gerstl, Eng, Hayward, Tavastjerna and Bond 1967; Rinne et al. 1970; Clausen and Hansen 1970; Gerstl, Eng, Tavastjerna, Smith and Kruse 1970). Studies dealing with the chemical neuropathology of multiple sclerosis have concentrated mainly on the analysis of lipids in white matter and purified myelin fractions. However on the basis of combined neurochemical and ultrastructural studies Rinne et al. (1970) came to the conclusion that early changes in MS possibly happen outside the myelin sheaths, especially in glia cells.

The results of the present study seem to support the conclusion drawn by Kurihara and Tsukada (1967, 1968) that phosphohydrolase is located mainly in myelin sheaths. The earlier results reported by Kurihara et al. (1969, 1970) and those of the present communication show that phosphohydrolase is a suitable indicator of demyelination. However, only in the present report has the phosphohydrolase activity been compared with myelin staining and cerebroside which are known as classical components of CNS myelin. Phosphohydrolase activities are higher than those reported earlier by Kurihara and Tsukada (1967, 1968), because a more complete liberation method including desoxycholate was used in the present study. Although the cerebroside analysis contains many sources of error its usefulness as an index of myelin seems to be unquestionable (Bass and Hess 1969). On the other hand one must accept that total glycolipids are included in the cerebroside values obtained by the method used in the present study. Nevertheless the proportion of sulphatide and gangliosides is low when compared with the total amount of cerebroside (Landolt and Hess 1966; Carter, Johnson and Weber 1965; Svennerholm and Svennerholm 1963). Cholesterol and cerebroside values are in accordance with the results reported by Einstein, Dalal and Csejtey (1970) in white matter outside plaques and plaque areas.

It is not known, at the membrane level, where phosphohydrolase is located in the myelin sheath e.g. in the major or intraperiodic line, and how it is bound to membrane. Although the molecular morphology of the myelin sheath is still poorly understood it is quite clear that basic protein, acid proteolipid and major proteolipid protein are main protein constituents of myelin (Mehl and Halaris 1970). However there seem to be some trace proteins in myelin and many are enzymatic proteins (Riekkinen et al. 1970; Rumsby, Riekkinen and Arstila 1970; Frey, Riekkinen, Rinne and Arstila 1970).

30

Our results do not suggest that phosphohydrolase is selectively attacked in the demyelination process and it can be envisioned that, as with decreased cerebroside values, it represents the gradual degradation of myelin lamellae. Quite opposite results have been reported for basic protein of myelin both in histochemical and bio-chemical studies (Hallpike, Adams and Bayliss 1970; Einstein *et al.* 1970; Riekkinen *et al.* 1970). These authors have shown that there is a selective loss of basic protein from myelin membrane in early myelin breakdown. On the other hand the cerebroside content of purified myelin fractions seems to be quite normal in MS and so the de-creased cerebroside values represent only the result of partial demyelination and the same may be argued for phosphohydrolase. For the understanding of the pathogenesis of multiple sclerosis the most important finding in the present communication is the increased activity of acid hydrolase in areas which showed normal or only moderately decreased values of cerebroside and phosphohydrolase. This result suggests that early lesions are outside the myelin sheaths and that demyelination, which is a characteristic feature of MS, is only a result of disease and not a primary disturbance in the disease process. If this observation is confirmed in later reports from other MS cases in au-topsy and also possibly in biopsy samples then the cause of the disease must be looked for somewhere else than in the myelin sheath (Field 1967; Jacob 1969). Although it may be an over-simplification, the discovery that early pathological change in MS is to be found in glial cells may suggest a situation analogous to SSPE, where the aetiology is a measles infection, but the pathogenesis of the disease remains an enigma.

REFERENCES

ADAMS, C. W. M., M. Z. M. IBRAHIM AND S. LEIBOWITZ (1965) Demyelination. In: C. W. M. ADAMS (Ed.), *Neurohistochemistry*, Elsevier, Amsterdam, pp. 437–487.

BADZIO, T. AND H. BOCZON (1966) The determination of free and esterified cholesterol in blood after separation by thin-layer chromatography, *Clin. chim. Acta*, 13: 794–797.

BANIK, N. L. AND A. N. DAVISON (1969) Enzyme activity and composition of myelin and subcellular frac-tions in the developing rat brain, *Biochem. J.*, 115: 1051–1062.

BARTLETT, G. R. (1959) Phosphorus assay in column chromatography, *J. biol. Chem.*, 234: 466–468.

BASS, N. H. AND H. HESS (1969) A comparison of cerebrosides, proteolipids, proteins and cholesterol as indices of myelin in the architecture of rat cerebrum, *J. Neurochem.*, 16: 731–750.

CARTER, E., P. JOHNSON AND E. WEBER (1965) Glycolipids, *Ann. Rev. Biochem.*, 34: 109–142.

CLAUSEN, J. AND I. B. HANSEN (1970) Myelin constituents of human central nervous system. Studies of phospholipids, glycolipids and fatty acid pattern in normal and multiple sclerosis brains, *Acta neurol. scand.*, 46: 1–17.

CUMINGS, J. N. (1955) Lipid chemistry of the brain in demyelinating diseases, *Brain*, 78: 554–563.

EINSTEIN, E. R., K. B. DALAL AND J. CSEJTEY (1970) Increased protease activity and changes in basic proteins and lipids in multiple sclerosis plaques, *J. neurol. Sci.*, 11: 109–121.

FIELD, E. J. (1967) The significance of astroglial hypertrophy in scrapie, kuru, multiple sclerosis and old age, together with a note on the possible nature of the scrapie agent, *Dtsch. Z. Nervenheilk.*, 192: 265–274.

FREY, H. J., P. J. RIEKKINEN, U. K. RINNE AND A. U. ARSTILA (1970) Peptidase activity of myelin during the myelination period in guinea-pig brain, *Brain Research*, 22: 243–248.

GERSTL, B., L. F. ENG, R. B. HAYMAN, M. G. TAVASTJERNA AND P. R. BOND (1967) On the composition of human myelin, *J. Neurochem.*, 14: 661–670.

GERSTL, B., L. F. ENG, M. TAVASTJERNA, J. K. SMITH AND S. L. KRUSE (1970) Lipids and proteins in multiple sclerosis white matter, *J. Neurochem.*, 17: 677–689.

HALLPIKE, J. F., C. W. M. ADAMS AND O. B. BAYLISS (1970) Histochemistry of myelin, Part 11 (Loss of basic protein in early myelin breakdown and multiple sclerosis plaques), *Histochem. J.*, 2: 323–328.

HESS, H. H. AND C. THALHEIMER (1965) Microassay of biochemical structural components in nervous tissue, Part 1 (Extraction and partition of lipids and assay of nucleic acids), *J. Neurochem.*, 12: 193–204.

JACOB, H. (1969) Tissue process in multiple sclerosis and para-infections and post-vaccinal encephalomyelitis. *Add. ad Int. Arch. Allergy*, 36: 22–34.

KURIHARA, T. AND Y. TSUKADA (1967) The regional and subcellular distribution of 2′,3′-cyclic nucleotide 3′-phosphohydrolase in the central nervous system, *J. Neurochem.*, 14: 1167–1174.

KURIHARA, T. AND Y. TSUKADA (1968) 2′,3′-Cyclic nucleotide 3′-phosphohydrolase in the developing chick brain and spinal cord, *J. Neurochem.*, 15: 827–832.

KURIHARA, T., J. L. NUSSBAUM AND P. MANDEL (1969) 2′,3′-Cyclic nucleotide phosphohydrolase in the brain of the Jimpy mouse, a mutant with deficient myelination, *Brain Research*, 13: 401–403.

KURIHARA, T., J. L. NUSSBAUM AND P. MANDEL (1970) 2′,3′-Cyclic nucleotide 3′-phosphohydrolase in brains of mutant mice with deficient myelination, *J. Neurochem.*, 17: 993–997.

LANDOLT, R. AND H. H. HESS (1966) Regional distribution of some chemical structural components of human nervous system, Part 2 (Cerebrosides, proteolipid proteins and residue proteins), *J. Neurochem.*, 13: 1453–1459.

LOWRY, O. H., N. J. ROSEBROUGH, A. L. FARR AND R. J. RANDALL (1951) Protein measurement with the Folin phenol reagent, *J. biol. Chem.*, 193: 265–275.

MEHL, E. AND A. HALARIS (1970) Stoichometric relation of protein components in cerebral myelin from different species, *J. Neurochem.*, 17: 659–668.

OLAFSON, R. W., G. I. DRUMMOND AND J. F. LEE (1969) Studies on 2′,3′-cyclic nucleotide-3′-phosphohydrolase from brain, *Canad. J. Biochem.*, 47: 961–966.

RIEKKINEN, P. J. AND J. CLAUSEN (1969) Proteinase activity of myelin, *Brain Research*, 15: 413–430.

RIEKKINEN, P. J., J. C. CLAUSEN AND A. U. ARSTILA (1970) Further studies on neutral proteinase activity of CNS myelin, *Brain Research*, 19: 213–227.

RIEKKINEN, P. J., J. PALO, A. U. ARSTILA, H. SAVOLAINEN, U. K. RINNE AND E. KIVALO (1970) Protein composition of multiple sclerosis myelin, *Arch. Neurol. (Chic.)*, In press.

RINNE, U. K., P. J. RIEKKINEN AND A. U. ARSTILA (1970) Biochemical and electron microscopic alterations in the white matter outside demyelinating plaques in multiple sclerosis. In: *Progress in Research and Therapy of Multiple Sclerosis*, In press.

RUMSBY, M. G., P. J. RIEKKINEN AND A. U. ARSTILA (1970) A critical evaluation of myelin purification. Non-specific esterase activity associated with central nerve myelin preparations, *Brain Research*, 24: 495–516.

SVANDBORG, A. AND L. SVENNERHOLM (1961) Plasma total lipid, cholesterol triglycerides and free fatty acids in a healthy scandinavian population, *Acta med. scand.*, 169: 43–49.

SVENNERHOLM, E. AND L. SVENNERHOLM (1963) The separation of neutral blood serum glycolipids by thin-layer chromatography. *Biochim. biophys. Acta (Amst.)*, 70: 432–441.

Protein Composition
of Multiple Sclerosis Myelin

Paavo J. Riekkinen, MD; Jorma Palo, MD; Antti U. Arstila, MD;
Heikki J. Savolainen; Urpo K. Rinne, MD; Erkki K. Kivalo, MD; and Harry Frey, MD

Numerous authors have shown that encephalitogenic protein is located in myelin but conflicting opinions have been expressed about the nature and structure of this protein. One group of workers' reported that the source of differing results is degradation of encephalitogenic protein during purification procedure. According to other investigators, however, microheterogeneity of myelin proteins also exists in vivo.

Under different experimental demyelinating conditions, the first step in myelin breakdown is early proteolysis of vulnerable protein components of myelin membrane. Histochemical studies have shown that this protein is the basic and possibly encephalitogenic constituent of myelin. The same authors reported that the amount of encephalitogenic protein decreases in areas of active demyelination process at the border of multiple sclerosis (MS) plaques. Although this decrease may not be involved in autoimmunization processes in central nervous system (CNS), it may well reflect general mechanism of early myelin breakdown. We would now like to report our own results of a study on the protein composition of purified myelin from normal human and MS white matter.

Material and Methods

Patients.—White matter samples taken at autopsy from seven patients with MS and from seven patients with no suspicion of MS or related diseases were analyzed. The diagnosis of MS was ascertained during life with all available clinical data and after death with histopathological examination. White matter samples from two MS patients were sent and also four other MS samples. One MS patient was from Finland. The American and Danish MS patients were autopsied within 9 to 12 hours after death, and the samples were kept frozen at −20 C prior to the analyses, also during transportation. The Finnish patient was kept after death at 4 C and autopsied after two days. The white matter samples were stored at −20 C until analyzed.

The ages of the MS patients varied from 36 years to 58 years and the ages of the control patients from 43 years to 64 years. Five of the MS patients were men and two were women. The corresponding figures for the control patients were two and four.

Dissection of Samples and Light Microscopy.—The material for chemical analysis was taken from macroscopically normal white matter at least 1 cm outside visible MS-plaques. The absence of plaques was ascertained by taking other half of each sample for light microscopic analysis. For this purpose the samples were embedded in paraffin and myelin sheaths stained with Luxol fast blue B. In none of the samples demyelinating plaques were found. No gliosis was seen in these areas. Numerous lymphocytes were seen in one MS sample but only a few or no foreign cells in other samples. The samples from control autopsies were taken from corresponding brain areas as the MS samples.

Purification of Myelin.—This was mainly according to the method published previously by Riekkinen and Rumsby in 1969.[8]

White matter dissected free from gray matter was rinsed in 0.32M sucrose to remove blood. It was then homogenized in 0.32M sucrose at pH 7.35 (10 millimoles of tromethamine hydrochloride buffer). After homogenization, nuclei and cell debris were removed by pelleting three times at 1,000 g for five minutes. The supernatant was rehomogenized after each pelleting. The final supernatant was spun down three times at 13,500 g for ten minutes. Each time the supernatant was discarded, and the sediment homogenized in the original volume in sucrose. The final pellet containing mitochondria and synaptosomes was called the crude myelin fraction. The next steps of purification consisted of successive isopycnic gradient centrifugations in 0.32M sucrose against 0.65M sucrose. The myelin layer was recovered each time between the two sucrose layers. Osmotic shock treatment was included between density gradient centrifugations. After each osmotic shock myelin was pelleted at 13,500 g for ten minutes.

Enzymic Assays.—The purity of the final myelin preparation was controlled every time with a series of enzymatic assays. Acid phosphatase served as a lysosomal marker, succinic dehydrogenase as a mitochondrial marker, lactic dehydrogenase as for soluble fraction, and peptidase as a marker for myelin.[9]

Electron Microscopy.—For quantitative morphometric analysis of myelin, the samples were fixed in a suspension of 0.1M sodium cacodylate buffered with 3% glutaraldehyde for three hours, washed and postfixed with 1% sodium cacodylate buffered with osmium tetroxide for one hour. The samples were then collected on filters (Millipore) and prepared for morphometry as described by Baudhuin and Berthet[10] and Frey et al.[11] The quantitative morphometrical analysis was done according to Frey et al.[11]

Protein Analysis.—Protein content of the myelin preparations was determined by the Lowry method.[12]

Electrophoretic Protein Analysis.—This was according to the method described by Mehl

and Halaris[13] using horizontal polyacrylamide (15%) gel, phenol-formic acid-water (14:3:3, W/V/V) solvent, and 1% solution of amido black in 7% acetic acid for fixation and staining of the proteins. The amount of protein most commonly pipetted from each sample was 10μg. The electrophoresis was carried out with a current of 10 ma for 30 minutes and then with 20 ma for 150 minutes. The gel was cooled with circulating tap water under the rack. The gel plates were destained with the same apparatus with a current of 60 ma and with 7% acetic acid as conducting medium as long as was necessary. Cytochrome C served as a marker during the electrophoresis. Scanning of the gel was performed with the aid of a microdensitometer (Canalco model E).

Results

Myelin Yield.—Myelin yield, as calculated on the basis of protein content, was from 18 to 25 mg with a starting material 10 gm of white matter (wet weight) in the control group, and from 10 to 15 mg in the MS group. The MS white matter thus seemed to contain less myelin than the normal white matter.

Purity of Myelin.—*Biochemical Studies.*—According to the enzymatic criteria (succinic dehydrogenase and acid phosphatase) for the purity of myelin preparations, the myelin was purified 150 to 250 times as compared to the original white matter. The values for peptidase, which were indicators for membrane enzymes, also were within very constant and acceptable limits.

Electron Microscopic Studies.—The quantitative morphometric analysis demonstrated that more than two thirds of the fraction were composed of compact myelin sheaths (69.6% ± 7.9%). The rest of the fraction was made up of smaller membrane fragments (29.1% ± 7.2%). All or at least the majority of these membranes were probably also derived from myelin sheaths. The axonal contamination was negligible (1.3% ± 0.2%) as was also the amount of clearly distinguishable organelles outside the myelin sheaths. Figure 1 is a typical example of an electron micrograph used for the morphometric analysis.

Protein Composition of Myelin.—The present electrophoretic system allowed analysis of all myelin proteins at the same time. A very characteristic and well reproducible pattern was obtained for all control samples (Fig 2). The pattern in control cases could be divided into three main portions as follows: (1) the most acidic proteins near the origin consisted of from five to six components; (2) the major proteolipid protein in the middle zone with two or three additional weak bands above it; and (3) the fastest moving and most basic protein which also was the strongest band in all normal samples. One or two faint components appeared above it when larger amounts of protein were applied to the gel. The first and second portions were identical in both the normal and MS samples. In MS myelin, however, only traces of the basic proteins could be observed (Fig 2). The sample was from an 88-year-old (number three in Fig 2, 3) woman who died from basilar thrombosis and pneumonia. In chemical analysis, increased levels of lysophosphatides were found in the same sample, possibly due to infarcts in brain tissue. In protein electrophoresis, the amount of basic protein was intermediate, ie, less than in the other controls but definitely more than in the MS patients (Fig 2, 1, 2, 4, and 8). The characteristic scanning patterns for MS and control samples are given in Fig 3. They confirm the clear-cut differences between the normal and MS patients.

Comment

Lipids have been studied in MS and other demyelinating diseases by a number of authors.[14-17] Except for some enzymes, little attention has been paid to CNS myelin proteins in MS.[18-20] Gerstl et al[21] could find no differences in soluble proteins in MS as compared to normal brains.

The present data seem to show that myelin yield is smaller from MS white matter or at least that the amount of myelin showing similar flotation properties with control myelin is decreased. This could mean either the existence of small predemyelinating lesions or changes in the composition of MS myelin which will result in some loss of myelin to other fractions. Our previous data, however, are more in favor of general changes in whole white matter.[22] Our bio-

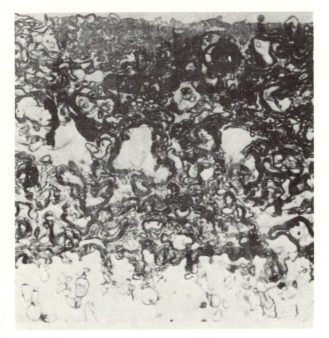

Fig 1.—Typical electron micrograph of myelin fraction collected on filter (Millipore) (× 15,000).

35

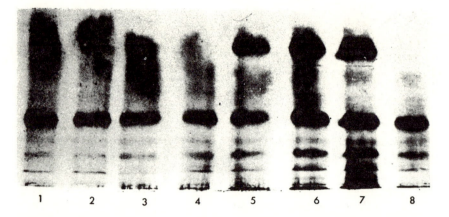

Fig 2.—Electrophoretic patterns of eight myelin samples run in same gel. Samples contained 15μg to 20μg protein. Numbers 1, 2, 4, and 8 are from MS cases. Number 5, 6, and 7 are from control cases which had died without any neurological disease. Case 3 was from 88-year-old woman who had thrombosis of basillary artery.

Fig 3.—Typical scanning curves for control (top) and MS (bottom) myelin samples (od indicates optical density of electropherogram). Note absence of major basic protein band from MS sample.

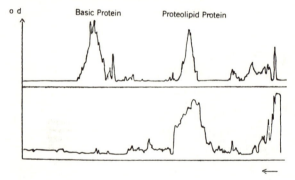

the other hand, Wolfgram et al[23] have postulated that the white matter in MS is normal.

Our results are in line with the findings by Moscarello et al[24] who analyzed myelin peptides of normal and MS cases. They found that one peptide was missing from the three MS samples as compared to the chromatographic pattern obtained from the normal samples.

The present electrophoretic system is very suitable for protein analysis, and the acidity of the solvent seems to exert no hydrolytic degradation on proteins. Although some artifacts can always be formed during electrophoretic runs, the effect should be identical in both the normal and MS samples. Autolysis of the white matter after death can be another source of error. It could be assumed that the loss of basic protein from the MS samples is due to this factor. The MS patients were autopsied, however, much sooner than control patients, except for the only Finnish patient. This patient showed the same typical MS pattern in protein electrophoresis thus proving that

chemical and electron microscopic data showed that the myelin separation was reproducible, and that the myelin preparations were well preserved and pure enough for accurate protein analysis.

Although many laboratories have been involved with the purification and chemical characterization of basic or encephalitogenic proteins, only few have analyzed it by histochemical methods. Hallpike and Adams[7] were able to show that the basic protein of myelin is the target of demyelinating process in peripheral nerve lesions. It may also be the first protein to disappear in MS. On the observed differences were not caused by autolytic processes.

Our findings together with some previous reports suggest that the basic or encephalitogenic protein is perhaps the first protein to be lost in any kind of myelin breakdown and thus the structural integrity of myelin membrane can no more be preserved. The case of the 88-year-old woman seems to indicate that this loss is not specific but may be due to various factors, including age The possibility cannot be excluded, of course, that the myelin proteins of MS patients are originally different from those of the normal people.

While biochemical investigations have shown that basic protein is involved in maturation of CNS myelin,[25,26] further studies are needed to show whether that protein has any role in the production of autoimmunization in MS[27] and if the disappearance is limited only to plaque areas.[28]

This investigation was supported by grants from the Finnish Research Council for Medical Sciences and Sigrid Jusélius Foundation.

Wallace W. Tourtellotte, MD, Ann Arbor, Mich, and Jorgen C. Clausen, MD, Copenhagen, provided the MS white matter samples, and Karin Lindberg gave technical assistance. The electron microscopic part of this study was done in the Laboratory of Electronmicroscopy at the University of Turku, Turku, Finland.

References

1. Nakao A, Davis WJ, Einstein ER: Basic proteins from the acidic extract of bovine spinal cord. Biochim Biophys Acta 130:163-179, 1966.

2. Einstein ER, Csejtey J: Degradation of encephalitogen by purified brain acid proteinase. Febs Letters 1:191-195, 1968.

3. Martenson RE, Deibler GE, Kies MW: Microheterogeneity of guinea pig myelin basic protein. J Biol Chem 244:4261-4267, 1969.

4. Hashim GA, Eylar EH: Allergic encephalomyelitis: Enzymatic degradation of the encephalitogenic basic protein from bovine spinal cord. Arch Biochem 129:635-644, 1969.

5. Eylar EH, Thompson M: Allergic encephalomyelitis: The physic-chemical properties of the basic protein encephalitogen from bovine spinal cord. Arch Biochem 129:468-479, 1969.

6. Eylar EH, Hashim GA: Allergic encephalomyelitis: Cleavage of the C-tryptophyl bond in the encephalitogenic basic protein from bovine myelin. Arch Biochem 131:215-222, 1969.

7. Hallpike JF, Adams CWM: Proteolysis and myelin breakdown: A review of recent histochemical and biochemical studies. J Hist Med 1:559-578, 1969.

8. Riekkinen PJ, Rumsby MG: Esterase activity in purified myelin preparations from beef brain. Brain Res 14:772-775, 1969.

9. Riekkinen PJ, Clausen J: Proteinase activity of myelin. Brain Res 15:413-430, 1969.

10. Baudhuin P, Berthet J: Electronmicroscopic examination of subcellular fractions: II. Quantitative analysis of mitochondrial population isolated from rat liver. J Cell Biol 35:631-648, 1967.

11. Frey HJ, Riekkinen PJ, Rinne UK, et al: Peptidase activity of myelin during the myelination period in guinea-pig brain. Brain Res 22:222-227, 1970.

12. Lowry OH, Rosebrough NJ, Farr AL, et al: Protein measurement with the folin phenol reagent. J Biol Chem 193:265-275, 1951.

13. Mehl E, Halaris A: Stoichiometric relation of protein components in cerebral myelin from different species. J Neurochem 17:659-668, 1970.

14. Gerstl B, Eng LF, Tavastsjerna M, et al: Lipids and proteins in multiple sclerosis white matter. J Neurochem 17:677-690, 1970.

15. Cumings JN, Goodwin H: Sphingolipids and phospholipids of myelin in multiple sclerosis. Lancet 21:664-665, 1968.

16. Amaducci LA, Artenoli G, Pazzagli A: Fatty acid and aldehyde changes in choline- and ethanolamine-containing phospholipids of white matter and erythrocytes occurring in multiple sclerosis, in Proceedings of Fourth International Congress of Neurological Surgery and Ninth International Congress of Neurology. No 193, Milano, Italy, Tamburini Editore, 1969.

17. Clausen J, Berg-Hansen L: Myelin constituents of human central nervous system. Acta Neurol Scand 46:1-17, 1970.

18. Lisak RP, Heinze RG, Falk GA, et al: Search for anti-encephalitogen antibody in human demyelinative diseases. Neurology 18:122, 1968.

19. Wolfgram F, Kotorii K: The composition of the myelin proteins of the central nervous system. J Neurochem 15:1281-1290, 1968.

20. Gerstl B, Eng LF, Hayman RB, et al: On the composition of human myelin. J Neurochem 14:661-670, 1967.

21. Gerstl B, Uyeda CT, Eng LF, et al: Soluble proteins in normal and diseased human brains. Neurology 19:1019-1026, 1969.

22. Rinne UK, Riekkinen PJ, Arstila AU: Biochemical and electron microscopic alterations in the white matter outside demyelinated plaques in multiple sclerosis. Prog Multiple Sclerosis Res, to be published.

23. Wolfgram F, Fewster ME, Mead JF: The amino acids and lipids of myelin in multiple sclerosis, in Proceedings of The Second International Congress for Neurochemistry. Milano, Italy, Tamburini Editore, 1969, pp 61-62.

24. Moscarello MA, Lowden JA, Wood DD: Polypeptides in cerebral myelin from normal humans and patients dying with multiple sclerosis. Neurology 18:295, 1968.

25. Einstein ER, Dalal KB, Csejtey J: Biochemical maturation of the central nervous system. Brain Res 18:35-49, 1970.

26. Gaitonde MK, Martenson RE: Metabolism of highly basic proteins of rat brain during postnatal development. J Neurochem 17:551-563, 1970.

27. Einstein ER: Problems related to the protein-eliciting experimental allergic encephalomyelitis, in Protein Metabolism of the Nervous System. New York, Plenum Press, 1970, pp 643-657.

28. Einstein ER, Dalal KB, Csejtey J: Increased protease activity and changes in basic proteins and lipids in multiple sclerosis plaques. J Neurol Sci 11:109-121, 1970.

ACID PROTEINASE ACTIVITY OF WHITE MATTER AND PLAQUES IN MULTIPLE SCLEROSIS

P. J. Riekkinen, J. Clausen, H. J. Frey, T. Fog and U. K. Rinne

Recent evidence suggests that lysosomal acid proteinase of neuronal and glial cells are involved in the pathogenesis of demyelination (*Hallpike et al.* 1969). These lysosomal enzymes of central nervous system (CNS) may, however, also originate from hematogenous cells (*Lampert* 1967).

Acid proteinase may liberate the basic protein from the myelin sheath (*Hallpike et al.* 1969). Furthermore, it is tempting to suggest that the liberated encephalitogenic protein could induce immunization in the extracerebral round cells and lymph modes (*Seitelberger* 1967). However, typical multiple sclerosis (MS) lesions contain, in the border-zone of plaques, only a small number of these inflammatory cells (*Périer & Gregoire* 1965, *Suzuki et al.* 1969). Therefore, at least in later stages of the disease, also cells originating from brain tissue may play a role in the autophagocytotic reactions.

Enzymic changes in MS brains occur mainly in the border-zone of active plaques (*Adams* 1965). As acid proteinase may play a major role in the provocation of autoimmunity of MS (*vide supra*) and as the enzymic changes cannot be quantitated by histochemical means, the present work therefore gives data on the topographic changes in total specific activities of acid proteinase of MS brains.

MATERIAL AND METHODS

Patient material: Autopsy samples were taken from 13 MS diagnosed as previously indicated (*Clausen et al.* 1969). All brains, by macroscopical examination, showed typical plaques. Only plaques with periventricular distribution were selected for enzymic studies. Three different samples were taken during visual inspection under a dissection microscope (1) from centre of plaques, (2) from border-zone of plaques, and (3) from corpus callosum outside of plaques. 11 brain autopsy specimens from corresponding topographic areas in patients dead of diseases without neurological symptoms were used as controls. One beef brain was obtained immediately after death from the Central Slaughter House of Copenhagen. This brain was used for evaluation of the effect of autolysis on activity of acid proteinase.

All the autopsy samples of MS and control patients were taken approximately 10–26 hours after death. Initial studies were made on the effect of autolysis on the activity of acid proteinase in beef brain. White matter from corpus callosum of this beef brain was isolated immediately after death. In agreement with the procedure for storing human bodies for patho-anatomical studies, the corpus callosum was stored for six hours at room temperature ($+24°$), and thereafter at $0°$. At the intervals 1, 4, 8, 24, and 48 hours after death, samples (100 mg wet weight) were taken for assay of proteinase activity.

Homogenization: Samples (100 mg wet weight) were homogenized in 1 ml distilled water for 3 minutes at 900 rpm in a teflon homogenizer (Thomas type A) with nine up-and-down passes of the pestle (temp $0°$).

Assay of acid proteinase: All the assays were performed on total homogenates to which was added 0.1 per cent (v/v) Triton-X-100 (alkyl-phenoxy-polyethoxy-ethanol, Rohm and Haas, Philadelphia, Pa, U.S.A.) 20 min prior to the assay. Denaturated human haemoglobin (Kabi AB, Stockholm, Sweden) was used as substrate according to the method described earlier (*Riekkinen & Clausen* 1969).

Protein determinations: They were made on total solubilized homogenate by means of the Biuret method as described by *Clausen* (1969).

Statistical methods: Student's t-test was used for the statistical evaluation of the results.

RESULTS

Initial studies on the effect of autolysis *in situ* (Table 1) revealed that no significant *post mortem* changes occur in the specific activities of acid proteinase. Therefore, the activities estimated in autopsy specimens are representative of the *in vitro* activities. The specific activity of the total homogenate made at zero-time also remained constant during two days' storage at $0°$ C.

Table 1. *Stability of acid proteinase of corpus callosum when specimens were stored first for six hours at room temperature (24° C) and then at $+4°$ C.*

	Storage of corpus callosum (mμmoles/mg prot/h)	Storage of fresh tissue homogenate of corpus callosum (0°) (mμmoles/mg prot/h)
1 hour	24.6	24.6
4 hours	23.1	27.1
8 hours	24.0	22.0
24 hours	24.0	26.5
48 hours	24.1	24.7

Table 2 gives the mean values for 13 autopsy samples in MS compared to those of 11 control cases. The centre of the plaque showed significantly lower specific activities than the control samples (P ≤ 0.001), and the values were also significantly lower in the centre of plaques than in border-zone of plaques (P ≤ 0.001). Here, the activity of acid proteinase was highest; thus the specific activities were higher than in white matter outside the border-zones (P ≤ 0.01). There was no significant difference between the white matter of control brains and the so-called normal white matter of MS brains.

Table 2. Mean values for acid proteinase of 13 MS brains. Specimens were taken from plaques, border-zones of plaques, and from macroscopically normal white matter. The data are compared to 11 control samples of corresponding brain areas. All values are presented in mμ moles/mg prot/hour at 37°. For experimental data see the text. The standard deviations are indicated.

1. Centre of plaque in MS brains	14.6 ± 2.8
2. Border-zone of plaque in MS brains	34.8 ± 7.6
3. White matter outside of plaques in MS brains	21.4 ± 2.1
4. Normal white matter; brain autopsy specimens of patients without neurological disease.	19.4 ± 2.6

DISCUSSION

In analysing enzymic activities of brain autopsy samples, the effect of autolysis on enzyme activities must be known. The present demonstration of the *in vivo* stability of acid proteinase corresponds to the *in vitro* studies of *Coffey & DeDuve* (1968). Also, other lysosomal hydrolases seem rather stable during storage (*Lundqvist & Öckerman* 1969).

Previously, histochemical methods have shown an increase in enzymic activities in border-zone of plaques in MS (reviewed by *Adams* 1965). These changes correspond to the findings that the myelin protein, in early stages of Wallerian degeneration, is sensitive to proteolysis (*Adams & Tuqan* 1961). The proteolysis, both in central and peripheral nerve myelin sheath, liberates pieces of the encephalitogenic protein (basic protein) (*Adams & Bayliss* 1968). This liberation may give rise to immunocompetent clones of lymphocytes being formed with immunospecificity against the basic protein. This event may cause an auto-immunization directed against the myelin sheath and thereby causing demyelination (*Adams & Hallpike* 1968).

The results obtained in the present study showed that acid proteinase activity increased during active demyelination, especially in the border-zone of plaques. Therefore, acid proteinase may play a primary or secondary role in the demyelination process as liberator of basic protein from the myelin sheath.

We are unable to demonstrate significant changes in the activity of acid proteinase in the so-called normal white matter of MS brains, where changes in lipid and/or fatty acid composition have been traced (*Gerstl et al.* 1965, *Cumings & Goodwin* 1968, *Clausen & Berg Hansen* 1970).

Recently, using a purification procedure for the elimination of proteinase inhibitors and other contaminating material before assay of proteinase activity, *Roboz Einstein* (1969) reported 3–4 times increased values for acid proteinase in normal white matter outside of plaques in MS brains. As there are multiple forms of acid proteinase in CNS (*Marks & Lajtha* 1965), the increased activity of purified acid proteinase may concern only one of these multiple forms of proteinases, which in an early stage of the disease reacts outside the demyelinating region. On the other hand, there can be a certain source of error in assaying prepurified proteinases after multiple steps of fractionation of the tissue homogenate, because we found that a part of the acid proteinase is denatured by the acetone often used for purification.

REFERENCES

Adams, C. W. M. (ed.) (1965): Neurochemistry. Elsevier Publ. Co., pp. 332–400.

Adams, C. W. M., & O. B. Bayliss (1968): Histochemistry of myelin. V. Trypsin-digestible and trypsin-resistant proteins. J. Histochem. Cytochem., *16*, 110–114.

Adams, C. W. M., & J. F. Hallpike (1968): Histochemistry of neuroglia and myelin breakdown. J. Neurol. Neurosurg. Psychiat., *32*, 162.

Adams, C. W. M., & N. A. Tuqan (1961): Histochemistry of myelin. II. Proteins, lipid-protein- dissociation and proteinase activity in Wallerian degeneration. J. Neurochem., *6*, 334–341.

Benetato, G., & E. Gabrielescu (1964): Histochemistry of Proteases in allergic reactions. Ann. Histochim. *9*, 295–304.

Clausen, J. (1969): The effect of vitamin A deficiency on myelination in the central nervous system of the rat. Europ. J. Biochem., *97*, 513–517.

41

Clausen, J., & I. Berg-Hansen (1970): Myelin constituents of human central nervous system. Studies of phospholipid, glycolipid and fatty acid pattern in normal and multiple sclerosis brains. Acta neurol. scand. *46*, 1–17.

Clausen, J., T. Fog & E. Roboz Einstein (1969): The clinical value of assaying proteins in the cerebrospinal fluid. Acta neurol. scand. *45*, 513–528.

Coffey, J. W., & C. DeDuve (1968): Digestive activity of lysosomes. I. The digestion of proteins by extracts of rat liver lysosomes. J. biol. Chem., *243*, 3255–3263.

Cumings, J. N., & H. Goodwin (1968): Sphingo-lipids and phospholipids of myelin in multiple sclerosis. Lancet, Sept. *21*, 664.

Gerstl, B., M. G. Tavaststjerna, R. B. Hayman, L. F. Eng & J. K. Smith (1965): Alteration in myelin fatty acids and plasmalogens in multiple sclerosis. Ann. N.Y. Acad. Sci. *122*, 405.

Hallpike, J. F., C. W. M. Adams & O. B. Bayliss (1969): Histochemistry of myelin. IX. Neutral and acid proteinases in early Wallerian degeneration. J. Histochem., 1969, in press.

Lampert, P. (1967): Electron microscopic studies on ordinary and hyperacute experimental allergic encephalomyelitis. Acta neuropath. (Berl.), *9*, 99–126.

Lundquist, A., & P. A. Öckerman (1969): Fine needle biopsy of the liver in healthy adults. Activity of lysosomal acid hydrolases. Enzym. biol. clin., *10*, 300–304.

Marks, N., & A. Lajtha (1965): Separation of acid and neutral proteinases of brain. Biochem. J., *97*, 74–83.

Périer, O., & A. Grégoire (1965): Electron microscopic features of multiple sclerosis lesions. Brain, *88*, 937.

Riekkinen, P. J., & J. Clausen (1969):Proteinase activity of myelin. Brain Res. *15*, 413–430.

Roboz Einstein, E. (1969): Paper read at the 2nd Int. Congr. Neurochem. Milan.

Seitelberger, F. (1967): Autoimmunologische Aspecte der Entmarkungsencephalitiden. Nervenartz, *38*, 525–535.

Suzuki, K., J. M. Andrews, J. M. Watlz & R. D. Terry (1969): Ultrastructural studies of Multiple Sclerosis. Lab. Invest., *20*, 444–454.

Multiple Sclerosis: Twenty Years on Low Fat Diet

Roy L. Swank, MD

Materials and Methods

Patient Material.—Evaluation and discussion of the materials and methods were presented in detail in a previous paper. The more pertinent points, however, will be included here. From December 1948 to April 1954, 264 patients with multiple sclerosis were examined at the Montreal Neurological Institute; 108 were seen only a few times. The remaining 156 patients maintained contact to and beyond April 1954, and no patients were added after this date. Two were rejected because of uncertain diagnosis, and eight were lost during the ensuing years. The remaining 146 patients are included in this report of progress to July 1, 1968. Most cases (72%) were diagnosed in the inpatient or outpatient services of the Montreal Neurological Institute; 22% were diagnosed by other qualified consultants in Veterans Administration Hospitals in Canada and northern New York State, and then referred to me. Six percent were seen and evaluated only by me.

An exacerbating-remitting course from onset with two or more episodes was required, with evidence from history and examination that the central nervous system had sustained lesions disseminated in time and space. This was clear in all but two cases in which initial relapses were followed by complete clinical remissions. A subsequent questionable relapse occurred in each case after which no further neurological signs or symptoms developed.

The distribution of patients in terms of neurological disability (Table 1), age at onset (Table 2), and duration of disease prior to diet (Table 3) are compared to other studies.

The neurological grades or rates used in the present study are as follows:

0 Normal performance and normal neurological examination results.

1 Normal physically and mentally; abnormal neurological signs present.

2 Actively ambulant, neurological signs present—usually working part-time or full-time.

3 Severely impaired performance; still ambulant—few working.

4 Wheel chair.

5 Bed.

6 Dead.

In our previous report, grades 4 and 5 were combined to form grade 4 alone and grade 5 was the dead category.

The patients were seen at two- and then four-week and later at three-month intervals. For the week preceding each visit, the patients recorded everything they ate. After July 1954 the patients were seen and examined once a year. Food intake records were sent to us every three months until the 15th year of the study. In the last five years this has been done yearly.

The Diet.—In the first years of the study (1948 to 1951) the diet contained 20 to 30 gm of fat daily, mostly from milk and animal sources. In 1951, butterfats were eliminated, animal fats were restricted to 15 gm daily and 10 to 15 gm *fluid* vegetable oils, and 5 gm cod liver oil were added to the daily diet. Corn oil, cottonseed oil, olive oil, peanut oil, soyabean oil, and safflower oil were included in the new oil supplement. Margarine, shortening, and hydrogenated peanut butter were disallowed. The diet contained a minimum of 50 gm and usually 60 to 90 gm of protein. Carbohydrates were consumed as required to make up the caloric need. One egg and several glasses of skim milk daily were recommended for their protein content. For animal protein intake, while avoiding additional fat contained in meat, patients were encouraged to eat fish three or more times a week. Most patients increased their fruit and vegetable intakes. Patients were instructed to measure all fat and oil-containing foods frequently to maintain a constant visual image of the prescribed allotments. For weighing, a small postal scale, and for volumetric measurements, standard measuring cups were used.

The "fractional fat" contained in small amounts in many foods, notably bread, was not included in the daily reckoning.[1-4] Careful analyses of total lipid intakes in the 1952 to 1954 period indicated that this averaged about 10 gm daily (Table 4). Estimated values for the intakes of the different food stuffs were determined from written records, not always accurate. Amounts were usually specified grossly, except in the matter of meats which were often weighed by the patient. Consequently, frequent errors and gross inaccuracies occurred. However, an averaging resulted from the frequent evaluations. It is these "averages" of fats and oils which we consider significant and which have been correlated with the course of the disease. *To the "average values" one must add the 10 gm of fractional fat to arrive at a more accurate estimate of the total fat intake.* In our opinion, the oil intakes as estimated are reasonably accurate.

We have defined *fats* as lipids solid at room temperature (70 F). In addition to butter and animal fat (lard), this includes all the margarines, hydrogenated oils other than margarine, ie, vegetable shortening (Crisco), chocolate, and hydrogenated peanut oil in peanut butter. *Oils* are fluid at room temperature, both those of vegetable and of fish (cod liver oil) origin. To avoid confusion due to labeling of many processed foods, patients were instructed not to use cake and other prepared mixes, nor other processed foods, unless we were first consulted, since hydrogenated oils are often labeled as "vegetable oil."

During the last 17 years of the study, the oil intake was substantially increased in many patients; in some, as much as 40 to 50 gm of oil was consumed daily during these years. Many others continued the diet originally prescribed. After 1952, we consistently encouraged patients to eat less than 15 gm of fat daily, but were not uniformly successful in accomplishing this.

We can be certain that the total lipid intakes were higher than indicated in previous papers,[1-4] yet substantially less than the patients had eaten before the study. Because total caloric intakes were low, averaging 1,788 for women and 2,164 for men, total lipid calories (fats plus oils) averaged 25% to 29% of the total. Calories from *fats* alone, however, averaged 15% to 17% of the total calorie intake, to which were added about the same number of calories from *oils*. In the last 17 years, the average intake of oil rose to as much as 50 gm daily in some patients. Simultaneously, fat intake decreased probably by an average of about 10 gm as the result of substitution of fish and sea food for meat.

Most patients lost weight because of the low caloric intake until they were thin by most

Table 1.—Patients in Each Neurological Grade Prior to Starting Low Fat Diet

Neurological Grade	No. (%) in Each Category		
	Swank	Allison[6]	VA[7]
0	1 (1)	1 (1)	0
1	27 (18)	5 (12)	2 (1)
2	61 (41)	8 (20)	48 (26)
3	44 (30)	9 (22)	54 (29)
4	12 (8)	3 (7)	50 (27)
5	1 (1)	14 (38)	30 (16)
Total cases	146	40	184

Table 2.—Ages at Onset of Multiple Sclerosis in Treated Cases

Age at Onset*	No.	%
<20	17	12
20-24.9	46	32
25-29.9	32	22
30-34.9	24	16
35-39.9	13	8
>40	14	9

* Average age at onset, 27.85 years.

standards. They were encouraged to remain lean, and were warned against gaining weight rapidly. Some patients, especially women, later regained part of the lost weight. To assist the patients, the low fat diet was published in book form.[8] At present, more than 1,000 patients are currently managing to follow the dietary regimen it outlines.

Of 146 patients approximately 80% or 118 adhered closely to the diet, as previously reported.[4] The others followed diet less well, and some poorly. In these, the fat intake was usually high, the oil intake low.

In 1954, the patient material was analyzed, and numerical evaluations were given for the neurological states (grade numbers) and the performance of the patients from the beginning of the study. Subsequently, the condition of the patient and his lipid intake were evaluated yearly. For the present study all pertinent data were recorded on cards for computer analysis. The entire experiment has been monitored by me and the diet evaluated by two observers.

Results

Exacerbation Rate.—*Prior to Low Fat Diet.*—The exacerbation rate (relapse per patient per year) probably varies from one population group to the other; it is necessary to determine this rate separately for each group of patients. Many observers consider minor events, lasting one day or less, as fluctuations, reserving "relapse," "exacerba-

Table 3.—*Duration of Disease Prior to Low Fat Diet or Observation in Allison's and VA Cases**

Duration of Disease Prior to Observation (yrs)	No. (%) in Each Category		
	Swank	Allison[6]	VA[7]
<1	28 (19)	3 (7)	...
1-2.9	25 (17)	3 (7)	57 (31)
3-4.9	27 (18)	3 (7)	...
5-9.9	31 (21)	9 (22)	64 (35)
>10	35 (24)	22 (60)	63 (34)
Total cases	146	40	184
Av duration of disease prior to observation	6.2	...	6.4

* Each VA figure includes those categories above it in the table for which details are not available.

tion," or "attack" for longer, more disabling events. Differences between the two categories are not clearly defined and lead to different interpretations of the same data by different observers. Patients may also forget events occurring a year or more before inquiry, and different techniques of data gathering may lead to widely divergent conclusions. Thygessen[9] questioned his patients at intervals averaging three weeks and so obtained the high rate of 1.2 relapses per patient per year. Müller[10] obtained his data from hospital records and found a low rate of only about 0.2 relapses per patient per year. Intermediate rates were arrived at by Alexander et al,[11] McAlpine and Compston,[12] and Compston.[13]

Careful questioning of the patients led to the following relapse rates for the three years prior to starting diet (Fig 1): 0.8 per patient per year the third year prior to inquiry, 0.8 per patient per year the second year prior to inquiry, and 1.3 per patient per year the year prior to inquiry.[4] Most patients came to us while in relapse and hence the rate for the year prior to inquiry was increased. Due to forgetfulness, the relapse rate was probably decreased in the second and third years prior to inquiry. Thus, in this series the prediet relapse rate was probably no lower than 0.8 nor higher than 1.3 per patient per year, with an estimated average rate of 1.0 per patient per year.

This rate is midway between that of Thygessen[9] (1.2 per patient per year) and Alexander et al[11] (0.75 per patient per year). Other rates found by Müller,[10] McAlpine and Compston,[12] and Compston[13] are significantly lower and probably reflect the

differences in history-taking techniques, material available to the investigator, and the diet (see "Comment"[14]).

Data While on Low Fat Diet.—In the 118 patients who carefully followed the low fat diet there was a sharp drop in relapse rate to about 0.3 per patient per year during the first year. During the next five years, a progressive decrease occurred to a low of 0.05 per patient per year. When the occasional "off diet" relapses were included in the evaluation, the relapse rate was only slightly greater (Fig 1). From the tenth year no correction was made for these few off diet relapses. Thus, there was a 70% decrease in relapse rate the first year, and a subsequent additonal decrease of 25% in the succeeding five years, a cumulative decrease of about 95%. Further, the relapse rate remained consistently near or below 0.05 per patient per year in the last 14 years of study.

The few relapses which occurred were very mild and of short duration, except when the patient went off diet, or following operations, pregnancy, or shock from bleeding. Patients were considered off diet when they consumed two to three times the allotted fat intake for more than two weeks.

Performance (Working Ability).—MacLean and Berkson[15] observed the survival rate of ability to work and to walk in 278 multiple sclerosis patients who were able to work and walk at their first visit. They suggested that this furnished "a minimal base line that a proposed therapeutic regimen must improve on before evidence for effectiveness can be accepted."

A strict comparison of their cases with mine is not possible because the interval between onset and arrival at the clinic for the 278 cases included in MacLean and Berkson's series is not known. For the entire 418 patients from which these 278 were selected, this interval averaged 7.0 years while for mine the interval averaged 6.2 years.

In the present report the analysis is extended to 16 years for my cases. Further, my cases are analyzed in two ways. First, those actually able to work and walk when first seen in the clinic (72 cases) are graphed separately (Fig 2, *dashed line*). Since 25 patients were unable to work or walk temporarily because of an exacerbation when first seen, those that remitted sufficiently to return to a working and walking state during the ensuing year were added to the first group (Fig 2, *dot-dashed line*).

These two additional analyses confirm the analysis of 1960[4] and indicate that all patients on diet did much better than the Mayo Clinic group.

Mortality.—When all 146 patients were considered, the average duration of observation was 17.1 years. Thirty-one or 21% were dead and 115 or 79% were still alive (Table 5). In these and in other studies, deaths from all causes were included. The average yearly death rate for my cases was 1.2%. A control group of the general population matched for age, sex, and duration of observation would have had an expected annual average death rate of 0.45%.

Other studies are summarized for comparison.[6,7,10,16,17] Allison's[6] cases were seen twice, in 1929 and again in 1949. The VA patients were seen after 1954. Duration and severity of disease were somewhat greater than in my cases at the beginning of the period of observation in both Allison's[6] and the VA patients (Table 1 and 3). Only the 129 cases of Müller's[10] group three were used, as Müller considered this group most representative. Müller's study was retrospective, the data obtained from hospital records.

Based on the number of expected deaths from actuarial tables, the death rate in the VA study was 11 times that expected; in the Müller series 4.5 times that expected; and in Swank's patients (all cases) 2.5 times the expected rate. In studies by Ipsen[16] and by Abb and Schaltenbrand[17] death rates were determined, but actuarial data were lacking (Table 5).

It was possible to correct for differences in duration (and perhaps also for severity) at the beginning of the period of observation by charting deaths against duration (Fig 3). There was a strikingly lower death rate (all causes) for my cases on low fat diet than for the other four groups. This difference is shown from the tenth year of disease. After more than 35 years of disease, 21% of my cases were dead; for the 118 good dieters reported before,[4] 19% were dead; of the 28 poor dieters, 29% were dead. Seventy percent of Allison's cases were dead at this time.

The death rate in untreated or ineffectively treated cases of multiple sclerosis was three to four times higher than in patients in this study maintained on a low fat diet for up to 20 years.

In a recent study Kurtzke et al[18] reported the survival rate of 762 veterans with multiple sclerosis who had had 90 days or more military service and who had received a diagnosis of multiple sclerosis in an army hospital between 1942 and 1951. Their Fig 1, showing survival rate for duration of disease up to 30 years, is shown in our Fig 4. For comparison, the survival rate of my cases for up to 35 years of disease, and for the VA study of approximately 14.4 years is included in our Fig 4. My cases exhibit a substantially higher rate of survival than either of the two groups of veterans. The difference in survival between the two groups of veterans raises some doubt concerning the validity of one or both groups, and this will be discussed later.

Course of Multiple Sclerosis in Untreated and Low Fat Diet-Treated Cases.—Scores of functional ability were surprisingly close and would indicate that the course of the disease in different groups of untreated pa-

Table 4.—Food Intakes When So-Called Invisible Lipids are Included

			Lipids (gm)			Total Calories
	Protein	Carbohydrate	Fat	Oil	Total	
Women (No. 42)						
High	119	486	47	58	97	2,915
Low	33	93	20	10	32	792
Av	81	240	34	22	56	1,788
Men (No. 27)						
High	149	469	57	39	85	2,800
Low	59	187	25	9	34	1,419
Av	100	302	38	22	61	2,164

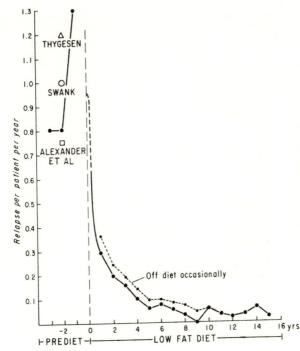

Fig 1.—Relapse rates before and during period on low fat diet. Only 118 patients who followed diet closely are included. Rates for each of three prediet years, based on history, and their average are charted. "Off diet occasionally" relapses attending dietary indiscretions by these patients are also included for first ten years; thereafter they are excluded. Average rates determined by Thygesen[9] and by Alexander[11] are charted in prediet period.

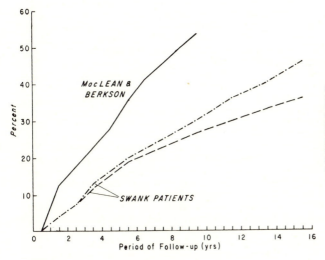

Fig 2.—Rate of decline of ability to work and walk. Dashed line includes all patients able to work and walk when first seen; dot-dashed line, those patients who were in relapse and unable to work when first seen, but in first year of treatment recovered to walk and work; solid line, corresponding data from MacL...a.i and Berkson.[15]

47

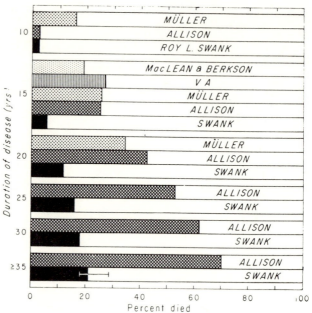

Fig 3.—Accumulated percentage of deaths from tenth year of disease for patients with multiple sclerosis. Figures for Müller are from Table 36 of his manuscript.[10] Figures for Allison's cases are determined from case histories.[6] Death rate for VA study was computed from 51 actual deaths in 184 patients followed up for an average of 6.4 years plus the average prestudy duration of disease which was 7.95 years from their Table 1.[7] Veterans Administration figure is an average for approximately 14.4 years after onset. Maximum-minimum symbol for my cases at ≥ 35 years indicates accumulated deaths at that time; death rates for poor dieters (28) and good dieters (118) are indicated in this column.

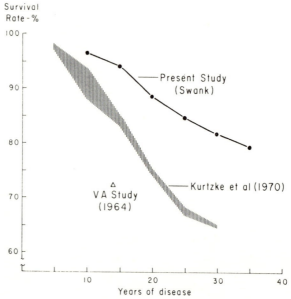

Fig 4.—Survival rates for years of disease. Curve for Swank's is from present study. Two groups of American veterans are also included in this graph—those by Kurtzke et al[19] and VA study.[7]

48

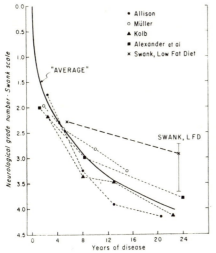

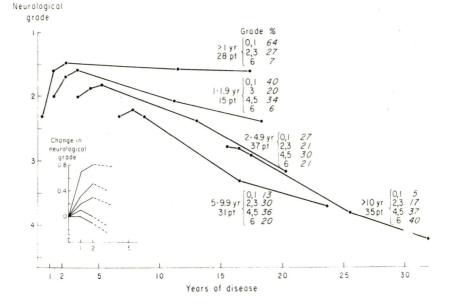

Fig 5.—Course of multiple sclerosis. Data for present curves were obtained from Allison's 40 cases,[9] Alexander et al's 554 cases estimated from trend of points shown in Fig 3 of his paper,[11] from Müller's data as calculated from Table 39 and 44 of his monograph,[10] and from an estimate of Kolb's data from Fig 5 of his paper.[1u] Their data were altered to conform to neurological ratings used in this paper. **Heavy line** indicates "average" curve; this line closely approximates hypothetical curve including all cases in my study presented in Fig 6 in a previous paper.[4] **Heavy dashed line** indicates treated cases, beginning 6.2 years after onset and ending 23.3 years after onset.

Fig 6.—Course of disease for patients with different durations of multiple sclerosis prior to low fat diet. **Solid lines** denote periods on diet for different groups; figures at right indicate number of patients in each group and percentage of patients in each grade at end of treatment period. **Insert** shows changes in grade based upon same data. Beginning neurological status is adjusted to 0 to show change in average neurological grade during first years of diet treatment. Duration of disease before diet is not charted.

49

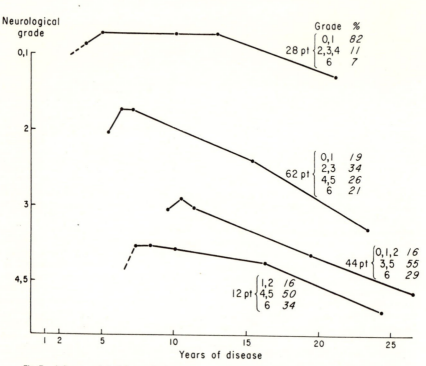

Fig 7.—Influence of initial neurological grade on course of disease in treated patients. **Dashed, then solid lines** indicate duration of disease and period on low fat diet. Figures at right indicate number of patients in each group and percentage in each grade at end of treatment period.

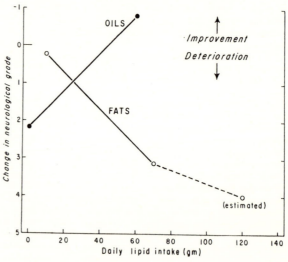

Fig 8.—Correlation of fat and oil intakes with neurological grade changes during 20 years of low fat diet, based on linear regression equation. **Dashed line** is hypothetical and based on assumption that average fat intake of untreated patients was 120 gm daily and that these patients would deteriorate to grade 4 in about 20 years (Fig 5).

Table 5.—Mortality for Treated Cases Compared to

Author	Av Years of Study	No. of Patients	No. of Deaths	No. of Expected Deaths From Life Tables	% Deaths per Year
Swank	17.1	146	31	11.25	1.20
Good diet*		118	23	...	1.10
Poor diet		28	8	...	1.70
Allison	20.0	40	28	...	3.50
VA	6.4	184	51	4.60	4.30
Müllert	20.0	129	...	...	2.70
Ipsen	...	784	...	...	3.98 male, 3.02 female
Abb and Schaltenbrand	5.0	958	240	...	5.00

* From previous paper.[4]
† Material 3.

tients is similar (Fig 5). The average change in neurological grade was from 2.3 to 4.0, a deterioration of 1.7 grades in 17 years beginning 6.2 years after onset of the disease. For the same period, patients on low fat diet deteriorated an average of 0.6 neurological grade, a significantly slower course. If only the 118 patients reported previously[4] who followed diet closely were charted separately, the average deterioration was even less—0.4 grade. The 28 patients who followed diet poorly deteriorated much faster, an average of 1.4 grades.

Factors Influencing the Course of Multiple Sclerosis During Low Fat Diet Treatment.—*Duration and Severity of Multiple Sclerosis Before Treatment.*—Early diagnosis and treatment are of utmost importance to prevent further progress of the disease with the low fat diet (Fig 6 and 7). The almost horizontal course of the disease after remission, during low fat diet treatment in patients whose conditions were diagnosed within one year of onset contrasts sharply with the steeper and almost parallel downward slopes for groups of patients whose diagnosis and treatment were delayed (Fig 6). Patients whose conditions were diagnosed within one year of onset of disease actually improved by 0.6 of a grade during the 20-year period of low fat diet treatment, whereas all others deteriorated; the deterioration increased as the duration of delay before diet increased. Patients with minimal involvement (grades 0 and 1) of multiple sclerosis when treatment was started also did very much better than those with more severe disease (Fig 7). An almost horizontal course from beginning to end of therapy was observed in patients with minimal neurologi-

cal involvement. A steeper and almost parallel rate of decline was observed in the other groups.

Early in the disease, remissions (initial rise in graph) were relatively complete, though not necessarily long (Fig 6, insert). As the duration of disease lengthened, remissions became less complete and finally failed to occur at all. This observation was possible because most patients came to our attention during an exacerbation. During the first few years of disease in untreated patients there was very rapid deterioration of neurological status (Fig 5). Patients on low fat diet tended to maintain their neurological status. However, few who had the disease for more than one or two years, or who, following remission, were already disabled, improved significantly.

Patients with minimal involvement (grades 0 and 1), who had also had symptoms less than one year when first seen, had a nearly 95% chance of remaining the same or improving during the 20 years of low fat diet (Table 6). In those with disease for 1 to 1.99 years the number of cases unchanged or improved dropped to approximately 75%, and for those with disease longer than two years it dropped further to about 50%. When patients moderately (grade 2) or severely (grade > 2) disabled were considered together, slightly less than 20% of the patients remained unchanged or improved at the end of the period. Also, in these more severely disabled patients the duration of disease prior to treatment had less influence on the course during treatment.

Influence of Lipid Intake on Course of Multiple Sclerosis.—Most patients followed our instructions well; others consumed sever-

Expected % Deaths per Year From Life Tables	Ratio of Actual Deaths to Expected Deaths Based on Life Tables
0.45	2.5:1
...	...
...	...
...	...
0.38	11:1
0.60	4.5:1
...	...
...	...

al times the suggested amounts of fats. The same variation occurred in the oil intake. Generally, though, high oil consumers were low fat consumers and vice versa. After an initial period of a few months, most patients developed eating habits which changed very little in subsequent years if periodically seen and diets evaluated. Since diets were evaluated more frequently in the first years of study, we averaged each patient's fat and oil intake for the first seven years of diet to arrive at the daily average fat and oil intake.

A linear regression equation was used to test the possibility of predicting changes in neurological grade as a function of fat and oil intakes. During the 20-year study, patients who consumed the least fat and the most oil deteriorated less than those who consumed more fat and less oil (Fig 8, *solid lines*).

Because low fat consumers were also the high oil consumers, it is not possible to conclude that a high oil intake improves the patient, although this may be true. It is clear, however, that a high oil intake was not harmful.

The conclusion that the low fat consumers did better during the 20-year period than those who consumed more fat was also borne out by clinical observation. Twenty-eight patients followed diet less well, yet consumed substantially less fat than before they went on the diet. Many of these 28 patients appeared to do well during the first 12 years of therapy, thereby raising the question of how low the fat level must be for maximum protection. In the last few years many of these patients deteriorated substantially. Patients who followed the diet care-

fully, however, continued to do very well (Fig 1, 2, 5, and 8). Therefore, for maximum protection, the diet needs to contain the minimal amount of fat recommended, possibly even less. I believe that a fat intake of 10 to 15 gm daily, exclusive of the 5 to 10 gm of fractional fat, should be the maximum allowed. In some instances we found it necessary to hold the fat intake below this level by substituting fish and sea food for meat. *These low levels of fat were possible only when the physician frequently reinforced the dieticians' instructions.* It was also found easier to maintain a very low fat intake when the oil intake was allowed to vary freely according to desire and caloric requirements.

Some General Clinical Observations.— During the first six months on the diet, relapses decreased in frequency and severity, but occasionally a severe relapse did occur. After the first year on the diet, severe relapses were very rare.

Fatigue, an outstanding symptom of disease in most cases, slowly lessened in patients on diet, and during the third year on diet seemed to improve substantially. However, a degree of fatigue with periodic spontaneous increases remained with patients regardless of how well they did. This could be intensified by too much activity, and was least marked in patients who started on diet early. Continuing deterioration to the point of complete disability in patients who carefully followed the low fat diet almost always was due to an intensification of signs and symptoms involving systems of the nervous system already involved; involvement of new, previously noninvolved systems or areas occurred rarely and was minimal.

During the first several years of therapy, patients were advised to rest (horizontally) for approximately one hour daily after lunch. They were also advised to get additional rest during periods of deep fatigue and to avoid nervous tension. Phenobarbital or butabarbital grains, ½ three times daily, was frequently prescribed. Overheating from sunlight or hot baths was warned against, and dark glasses were prescribed for bright light or sunlight for patients with visual troubles.

Transfusions immediately after major operations and childbirth have been recom-

52

Table 6.—Relationship of Duration and Severity of Multiple Sclerosis to Results of Therapy

Initial Neurological Rating	Years of Multiple Sclerosis Before Low Fat Diet	Neurological Grade 20 Yrs on Low Fat Diet			Same or Improved	Worse	Av Neurological Grade 20 Yrs on Low Fat Diet
		0-1	2	>2			
0-1	<1	18	0	1	18	1	0.77
	1-1.99	6	0	2	6	2	1.25
	2-5	9	3	7	9	10	2.05
	>5	4	1	3	4	4	2.00
	Total	37	4	13	37	17	
2	<1	0	1	3	1	3	3.00
	1-1.99	0	1	1	1	1	2.50
	2-5	0	1	8	1	8	4.10
	>5	1	5	16	6	16	3.60
	Total	1	8	28	9	28	
>2	<1	1	0	2	1	2	3.33
	1-1.99	0	0	5	5	0	4.00
	2-5	0	1	10	1	10	4.54
	>5	1	0	34	1	34	4.09
	Total	2	1	51	8	46	

mended routinely in the past 15 years, and this procedure has been used occasionally with apparent gratifying results in patients suffering from severe exacerbations.[20]

Comment

The criteria used in this study indicate that the course of multiple sclerosis patients on low fat diet was smoother and much less rapidly progressive than in untreated controls from the literature. A remarkable reduction in frequency and severity of exacerbations, a greatly reduced rate of loss of ability to walk and work, and a remarkably reduced death rate occurred in patients on the low fat diet. If the low fat-treated patients and the untreated patients with which they were compared were similar in all respects when first observed, the conclusion that the low fat diet was beneficial would be unavoidable.

Unfortunately this assumption cannot be made. Our own analyses have shown that Allison's patients and the Veterans Administration group of patients were more severely disabled than the low fat diet-treated patients when first seen (Table 1 and 3). There is no way of knowing exactly how Berkson and MacLean's patients compared with my patients except that in both groups, the patients were walking and working when first seen. Some of the resulting dilemma is dispelled by the length of this study. If duration and severity of disease were determining factors, one would have expected accelerated rates of deterioration to occur in my cases. This did not occur.

When considering the death rate, it was possible to correct for the longer observation in the untreated control patients by determining the death rates in relation to total duration of disease. This comparison also showed that treated cases did remarkably better than the other available groups. Unfortunately, there is no way to evaluate the inherent difference in the potential severity of disease in patients when first seen. The large number of patients, the duration of this study, and the very small loss of patients to the study (less than 6%) are significant.

It would also appear that the survival rate in low fat diet treated cases was far better than in the best of the nontreated cases so far published (Fig 4). There is concern, however, about the very different survival rates for the two groups of veterans, the VA group[7] and the Kurtzke et al group.[19] One can only speculate which of these patients more nearly represented the expected survival rate of young American men. The survival rates at approximately 15 years of disease for the VA group,[7] the patients of Allison,[6] of Müller,[10] and Ipsen,[16] computed from their death rates were similar; the computed rate for the VA group[7] is charted as a single point in Fig 4. This renders

53

suspect the later more optimistic survival rate[19] which is also charted in Fig 4. Severe and continuous nervous tension, a frequent accompaniment of military life, has a deleterious effect on multiple sclerosis. Perhaps the conditions for selection (90 days of military service and a diagnosis in an army hospital) by virtue of this tension precipitated multiple sclerosis in a number of patients who otherwise would not have developed it in a clinically recognized form, or would have developed it much later. After discharge from the army and release from the stresses of army life, the disease in these patients might be expected to pursue a relatively mild course.

It is still possible to argue that the 108 patients who were seen only a few times and then lost to the study were destined to be the more acutely ill. Such a claim seems unlikely, and experience in recent years has shown that many, if not most, of the patients who left the study, were those doing well. This has also been true of the more than 800 patients not included in this study seen during the past 15 years in Portland, Ore.

When all of these factors are considered, the conclusion that the low fat diet was significantly beneficial to the patients seems inescapable. There are very little data in the literature other than our study that confirm this conclusion, but data consistent with it are available. An early survey by Ackerman[21] showed marked variations in the geographic prevalence of multiple sclerosis in Switzerland. In the northern German-speaking cantons, the prevalence of multiple sclerosis was high, while only a short distance south in the Italian-speaking cantons, it was low. In the French-speaking areas an intermediate prevalence predominated. Recently, the distribution of cases was found to be little changed.[22] Gram[23] and Hvllested[24] noted marked variations in the prevalence of multiple sclerosis in different districts of Denmark, and similar geographic differences were shown in Norway,[25,26] Sweden,[27] and Scotland.[28]

Since there is a tendency for the prevalence of multiple sclerosis to be higher in the northern than in the southern part of the northern hemisphere, many students have held to the notion that latitude is important.

A number of studies appear to disprove this. Swank et al[25] found a very low prevalence of multiple sclerosis along the entire coast of Norway from the Arctic Circel to the temperate zone, a latitude spread of about 13°. A similar latitude spread with very low incidence of multiple sclerosis was also found in Japan.[29] On the other hand, in Switzerland,[21,22] marked geographic variations in prevalence were observed in neighboring areas, and in Israel[30,31] similar variations, based more on cultural differences, were found. The entire latitude spread of the populated portion of these countries is little more than 2°. In Norway[25] differences as great as eight to one in the prevalence of multiple sclerosis existed between coastal and central areas at the same latitude. One fact stands out. The prevalence and incidence of multiple sclerosis varies geographically. In all probability latitude is not the determining factor. Kurtzke[32,33] arrived at the same conclusion. The suggestion that the frequency of multiple sclerosis is related to geomagnetic effects[34] appears to be invalidated by the same data.

Because the average fat intake is high in countries having a high prevalence of multiple sclerosis and low in countries with few multiple sclerosis cases, I suggested in 1950[35] that the high incidence of multiple sclerosis in the more northern areas was due to the high fat intake of the general population. This suggestion was supported by the observation that the prevalence of multiple sclerosis seemed to vary directly with changes in the fat intake in occupied countries during World War II. In Norway the prevalence and incidence of multiple sclerosis in different districts varied directly with fat intake.[25] In Switzerland, the German Swiss have a high fat intake[36] and also a high prevalence of multiple sclerosis. More recently a similar relationship of fat intake to the prevalence of disease has been shown in Israel. Brunner and Löbl[37] found that the European Jews eat much more fat than the Yemenite Jews. European Jews have a high prevalence of multiple sclerosis, whereas the Yemenite Jews have a very low prevalence.[30] Indeed, Rozanski[31] stated that multiple sclerosis "seems to be unknown among the Yemenite Jews." In the northern part of the United States, one of the highest fat consuming areas of the world,[38] the incidence of multiple sclerosis is very high; whereas China,[39] Japan,[29] and Korea,[40] at a similar latitude, have extremely few cases of multiple sclerosis, and their people consume very little fat.[38] Grashchenkov et al[41] noted the general relationship of multiple sclerosis to latitude, but also stated that multiple sclerosis in Russia has the lowest frequency in areas where fruits and vegetables make up a substantial portion of the daily food intake. These arguments do not prove our hypothesis, but are consistent with it.

The low fat diet can be said to alter the course of multiple sclerosis from an exacerbating-remitting disease to a slowly progressive disease. When treatment was started early, the progress was very slow, and in many cases no deterioration other than that related to aging was evident in 20 years. In those in whom treatment was started late, the story was quite different; the course was smooth with few relapses, but visibly downhill.

It can be argued that our early cases who did so well on low fat diet represent those cases who had one attack and no more. MacKay and Hirano[42] were able to identify very few of these, and Lehoczky and Halasy-Lehoczky[43] estimated that perhaps about 4% of their 2,000 cases fell into these categories. It seems unlikely that we could have gathered together a large enough number of these long spontaneous remission cases to account for the benefits which we observed in patients on low fat diet. Only two of our cases had only one exacerbation.

It can further be argued from a long-term follow-up study by McAlpine[44] that there can normally be expected to occur a significantly large enough number of benign cases to explain our results. In McAlpine's 241 patients followed up for an average of about 20 years, who had prior multiple sclerosis less than three years, and who were able to work, 34% died, 33% were disabled, and 32% were still able to work. Fewer of these cases were unable to work and walk than were observed by MacLean and Berkson,[15] but more than in our treated cases (Fig 2). The deaths in McAlpine's series were about triple the death rate in our cases, yet less than in some of the other control series. These estimates suggest that Mc-

Alpine's cases did somewhat better both with regard to maintaining "normal" activity and to remaining alive than other untreated cases, but also significantly less well than the present series of treated patients. *McAlpine's cases had the advantage of significant fat deprivation during and after World War II—a period of about ten years from 1940 to 1950.*[14]

The mechanism by which the low fat diet alters the course of multiple sclerosis remains obscure. It is suggested that a fundamental cause of multiple sclerosis is a failure of fat transport in the blood of patients who have inherited, or otherwise acquired, a metabolic or other deficit incompatible with a high fat transport in the blood. The blood is essentially water in which carbohydrates and protein are dissolved. Fats are largely transported in the blood as an emulsion, maintained by surface active substances. It is suggested that the chylomicra and all other particulate matter in the blood (red and white cells and platelets) compete for these surface active substances, a deficiency of which leads to dense aggregation of red cells, the so-called sludging of Knisely et al.[45] Swank and Cullen[46,47] showed that intravascular aggregation of blood cells occurs in animals after large fat meals, a phenomenon subsequently observed in other animals[48,49] and in man.[50,51] Swank and Nakamura[52] also showed that this change in the circulation was accompanied by a reduction in oxygen availability in the brain and by convulsions and electrocardiographic changes in hamsters.[53,54] Oils either did not produce these changes or the changes were much less marked. More recently, Lino et al (unpublished data) observed in hamsters, dogs, and monkeys that ingested butter fat, lard, and margarine are transported in the blood largely in the red cell mass. The oils are transported primarily in the plasma. It is conceivable that the attraction of the fats for red cells after a large fat meal is fundamental to the development of multiple sclerosis. So-called sludging, observed in multiple sclerosis by Roizin et al,[55] a reduction in oxygen availability in brain tissues, and an increased permeability of the microcirculation[56] of the brain are possible steps in the genesis of the disease.[55] The increased vascular permeability theoretically would allow toxic surface active materials to invade brain tissues and unwrap myelin sheaths. Demyelinization and plaque formation would result.[58]

In another study of diet in multiple sclerosis, Evers[59] used what is essentially a raw or nonprocessed food diet. This diet, which contains many raw vegetables and fruits, has attracted attention in Germany. It is a reduced fat diet since meat and other cooked sources of fat are not allowed. Schuppien[60] claims that his patients do well on the Evers diet, but it is difficult from his publication to evaluate its success.

An untreated control was attempted early in this study. The control subjects quickly realized that a diet was under test and gradually reduced their own fat intake. It was then realized that it would be very difficult for one investigator to randomize patients and maintain the two groups on basically different diets for a significant period. Our correlation of fat intake with progress of the disease over a 20-year period is a type of control, although not as satisfactory as a randomized control. Aside from this we have been limited to a comparison of our own patients with other groups in the literature. The shortcomings of this type of control are well known.

This investigation was supported initially by the Multiple Sclerosis Society of Canada and later by Public Health Service grant NB 1536, the Multiple Sclerosis Society of Portland, Ore, and private donors.

Quentin D. Clarkson, PhD, gave assistance in analysis of the data. He is not, however, responsible for its interpretation. Aagot Grimsgaard and Kathleen H. Prichard maintained control and a record of the dietary intakes of the patients. The staff of the Montreal Neurological Institute made possible the yearly follow up of the patients.

References

1. Swank RL: Treatment of multiple sclerosis with low fat diet. *Arch Neurol Psychiat* 69:91-103, 1953.

2. Swank RL: Treatment of multiple sclerosis with low fat diet. *Arch Neurol Psychiat* 73:631-644, 1955.

3. Swank RL: Treatment of multiple sclerosis with low fat diet: Results of seven years' experience. *Ann Intern Med* 45:812-824, 1956.

4. Swank RL, Bourdillon RB: Multiple sclerosis: Assessment of treatment with a modified low fat diet. *J Nerv Ment Dis* 131:468-488, 1960.

5. Zeller RW: Ocular findings in the remission phase of multiple sclerosis. *Amer J Ophthal* 64:767-772, 1967.

6. Allison RS: Survival in disseminated sclerosis: A clinical study of a series of cases first seen twenty years ago. *Brain* 73:103-120, 1950.

7. Veterans Administration Multiple Sclerosis Study Group: Five-year follow-up on multiple sclerosis. *Arch Neurol* 11:583-592, 1964.

8. Swank RL, Grimsgaard A: *Low Fat Diet: Reasons, Rules and Recipes.* Eugene, Ore, University of Oregon Books, 1959.

9. Thygesen P: *The Course of Disseminated Sclerosis.* Copenhagen, Rosenkilde and Bagger, 1953.

10. Müller R: Studies on disseminated sclerosis. *Acta Med Scand* 222(suppl):1-214, 1949.

11. Alexander L, Berkeley AW, Alexander AM: Prognosis and treatment of multiple sclerosis—quantitative nosometric study. *JAMA* 166:1943-1949, 1949, 1958.

12. McAlpine D, Compston N: Some aspects of the natural history of disseminated sclerosis. *Quart J Med* 21:135-167, 1952.

13. Compston ND: Disseminated sclerosis: Assessment of effect of treatment on course of disease. *Lancet* 2:271-275, 1953.

14. Drummond JC: The Englishman's food today. *Practitioner* 160:3-12, 1948.

15. MacLean AR, Berkson J: Mortality and disability in multiple sclerosis. *JAMA* 146:1367-1369, 1951.

16. Ipsen J: Life expectancy and probable disability in multiple sclerosis. *New Eng J Med* 243:909-913, 1950.

17. Abb L, Schaltenbrand G: Statistsche Untersuchungen zum Problem der Multiplen Sklerose. *Deutsch Z Nervenheilk* 174:199 218, 1956.

18. Kurtzke JF, Beebe GW, Nagler B, et al: Studies on the natural history of multiple sclerosis. *Arch Neurol* 22:215-225, 1970.

19. Kolb LC: The social significance of multiple sclerosis. *Res Publ Assoc Res Nerv Ment Dis* 28:28-44, 1950.

20. Alexander L, Loman J, Lesses MF, et al: Blood and plasma transfusions in multiple sclerosis. *Assoc Res Nerv Ment Dis* 28:178-200, 1950.

21. Ackerman A: Die Multiple Sklerose in der Schweiz. *Schweiz Med Wschr* 61:1245-1250, 1931.

22. Georgie F, Hall P: Studies on multiple sclerosis frequency in Switzerland and East Africa. *Acta Psychiat Neurol Scand* 35(suppl 147):75-84, 1960.

23. Gram HC: Den disseminerede skleroses forekomst i Danmark. *Ugeskr Laeg* 96:823-825, 1934.

24. Hyllested K: Disseminated sclerosis in Denmark, thesis. Copenhagen, 1956.

25. Swank RL, Lerstad O, Strøm A, et al: Multiple sclerosis in rural Norway: Its geographic and occupational incidence in relation to nutrition. *New Eng J Med* 246:721-728, 1952.

26. Presthus J: Report on the multiple sclerosis investigations in West Norway. *Acta Psychiat Neurol Scand* 35(suppl 147):88-92, 1960.

27. Sallstrom T: Das Vorkommen und die Verbreitung der Multiplen Sklerose in Schweden: Zur geographischen Pathologie der Multiplen Sklerose. *Acta Med Scand* 137(suppl):1-141, 1942.

28. Sutherland JM: Observations on the prevalence of multiple sclerosis in northern Scotland. *Brain* 79:635-654, 1956.

29. Okinaka S, McAlpine D, Muyagawa K, et al: Multiple sclerosis in northern and southern Japan. *World Neurol* 1:22-38, 1960.

30. Alter M, Halpern L, Kurland LT, et al:

Multiple sclerosis in Israel: Prevalence among immigrants and native inhabitants. *Arch Neurol* 7:253-263, 1962.

31. Rozanski J: Contribution to incidence of multiple sclerosis among Jews in Israel. *Mischr Psychiat Neurol* 123:65-72, 1952.

32. Kurtzke JF: An evaluation of the geographic distribution of multiple sclerosis. *Acta Neurol Scand* 42:(suppl 19):91-117, 1966.

33. Kurtzke JF: A Fennoscandian focus of multiple sclerosis. *Neurology* 18:16-20, 1968.

34. Barlow JS: Correlation of the geographic distribution of multiple sclerosis with cosmic-ray intensities. *Acta Psychiat Neurol Scand* 35(suppl 147):108-131, 1960.

35. Swank RL: Multiple sclerosis: A correlation of its incidence with dietary fat. *Amer J Med Sci* 220:421-430, 1950.

36. Demole M: Alimentation militaire 1942. *Schweiz Med Wschr* 73:827-831, 1943.

37. Brunner D, Löbl K: Serum cholesterol. Electrophoretic lipid pattern, diet and coronary artery disease: A study in coronary patients and in healthy men of different origin and occupations in Israel. *Ann Intern Med* 49:732-750, 1959.

38. The state of food and agriculture—1948; A survey of world conditions and prospects. Washington, DC, Food and Agriculture Organization of the United Nations, September 1948.

39. Liu Tao-Kuan, Han Chung-Yen, Yen Ho Chün, et al: Multiple sclerosis: Report of five cases. *Chin J Neurol Psychiat* 4:137-142, 1958.

40. Kurtzke JF, Park CS, Oh J: Multiple sclerosis in Korea: Clinical features and prevalence. *J Neurol Sci* 6:463-481, 1968.

41. Grashchenkov BM, Hekht BM, Rogover AB, et al: Characteristics of the geographical distribution of disseminated sclerosis in the Soviet Union. *Acta Psychiat Neurol Scand* 35(suppl 147):148-158, 1960.

42. Mackay RP, Hirano A: Forms of benign multiple sclerosis. *Arch Neurol* 17:588, 1967.

43. Lehoczky T, Halasy-Lehoczky M: Forme 'bénigne" de la sclérose en plaques. *Presse Med* 71:2294-2296, 1963.

44. McAlpine D: The benign form of multiple sclerosis: Result of a long-term study. *Brit Med J* 2:1029-1032, 1964.

45. Knisely MH, Block EH, Elliot TS, et al: Sludged blood. *Science* 106:431, 1947.

46. Swank RL, Cullen CF: Circulatory changes in the hamster's check pouch associated with alimentary lipemia. *Proc Soc Exp Biol Med* 82:381-384, 1953.

47. Cullen CF, Swank RL: Intravascular aggregation and adhesiveness of the blood elements associated with alimentary lipemia and injections of large molecular substances: Effect on blood-brain barrier. *Circulation* 9:335-346, 1954.

48. Meyer JS, Waltz AG: Effects of changes in composition of blood plasma on pial blood flow. *Neurology* 9:728-740, 1959.

49. Swank RL: Changes in blood of dogs and rabbits by high fat intake. *Amer J Physiol* 196:473-477, 1959.

50. Harders H: Neue Beobachtungen zum Diätfehler. *Deutsch Ges Med* 62:499, 1956.

51. Williams AV, Higginbotham AC, Knisely MH: Increased blood cell agglutination following ingestion of fat, a factor contributing to cardiac ischemia, coronary insufficiency, and anginal pain. *Angiology* 8:29-40, 1957.

52. Swank RL, Nakamura H: Oxygen availability in brain tissues after lipid meals. *Amer J Physiol* 198:217-220, 1960.

53. Nakamura H, Swank RL: Electrocardiogram in hamsters after large fat meals. *Proc Soc Exp Biol Med* 105:195-197, 1960.

54. Swank RL, Nakamura H: Convulsions in hamsters after cream meals. *Arch Neurol* 3:594-600, 1960.

55. Roizin L, Abell RG, Winn J: Preliminary studies of sludged blood in multiple sclerosis. *Neurology* 3:250-260, 1953.

56. Broman T: Supravital analysis of disorders in the cerebral vascular permeability: II. Two cases of multiple sclerosis. *Acta Psychiat Neurol* 46(suppl): 58-71, 1947.

57. Swank RL: Treatment of multiple sclerosis with low-fat diet. *Arch Neurol Psychiat* 73:631-644, 1955.

58. Swank RL: *A Biochemical Basis of Multiple Sclerosis.* Springfield, Ill, Charles C Thomas Publisher, 1961.

59. Evers J: *Meine Therapie der Multiplen Sklerose.* Monatskurse ärztl. Fortbildung, 1954/5.

60. Schuppien W: *Die Evers-Diät.* Stuttgart, Germany, Hippokrates-Verlag, 1955.

Fluorescent Protein Tracing in Multiple Sclerosis Brain Tissue

John F. Simpson, MD; Wallace W. Tourtellotte, MD, PhD; Emre Kokmen, MD;
Julius A. Parker, MS; and Hideo H. Itabashi, MD

SIXTY to seventy percent of patients with multiple sclerosis (MS) have an elevated cerebrospinal fluid (CSF) immunoglobulin-G (IgG) in the presence of normal serum IgG.[1,2] These results prompted Kabat et al[1] to suggest that IgG was synthesized in the brain. The results obtained by Frick and Scheid-Seydel,[3] utilizing intravenous perfusion of radioactive IgG and albumin in a variety of patients, also suggested that the elevated CSF IgG in MS patients was derived from brain tissue or its coverings.

Recently we reported[4] for the first time that a positive correlation existed between the concentration of IgG in MS brain tissue (plaques of demyelination and surrounding normal-appearing white matter) and the IgG content of the CSF. In subsequent reports[5,6] we suggested that the IgG in MS brain tissue was synthesized in the brain rather than derived from the blood because the blood-brain barrier appeared to be intact to smaller molecules (albumin and bromide). Furthermore, it appears from a correlative study of the histology and IgG concentration in adjacent sections that IgG was synthesized by perivascular mononuclear cells or cells in the plaque, especially at its margin,[7] or both. We have also suggested[5,6] that the increased IgG in the normal-appearing white matter was the result of diffusion of IgG from areas of synthesis.

In this report we have attempted to localize more precisely the sites of synthesis of IgG in MS brain tissue. The IgG and albumin distribution was estimated by inspection of immunofluorescence in frozen-dried sections after incubation with fluorescein-conjugated antibody reagents. The pattern of distribution of specific fluorescence in and about MS plaque tissue was studied with respect to discernible histology as well as the histology revealed by hematoxylin and eosin-stained adjacent sections.

Materials and Methods

In an effort to minimize the loss of IgG from the tissue specimens, only quick-frozen unfixed tissues were employed. Antibody reagents of known titer were used to ensure antibody excess, since the general range of concentration of IgG and albumin in the tissues studied was known beforehand (166 to 524 mg/kg). Fifteen specimens from seven MS brains, all including plaque and surrounding normal-appearing white matter, and specimens from brains of patients with cerebral infarction, Guillain-Barré syndrome, uremia, and Creutzfeldt-Jakob disease, and three brains from patients without clinical or pathological evidence of brain disease were analyzed. Tissue specimens 1.5 cm in diameter were dissected from quick-frozen

(−90 C) 3-mm coronal brain slices, mounted, and allowed to warm to −15 C in a cryostat. Ten-micron sections were mounted on glass slides, thawed quickly, and dried at room temperature for one to two hours. The first and last sections were used for histologic evaluation.

Rabbit antihuman IgG conjugated with fluorescein isothiocyanate, unconjugated rabbit antihuman IgG, and conjugated rabbit antihuman albumin were obtained commercially. (To titrate the antibody content of the reagent, we used the method recommended by Kabat and Mayer.[8] The antibody titers were 2.2 mg/ml [anti-IgG] and 0.2 mg/ml [antialbumin].) Absorption of specific antibody from conjugated antihuman IgG serum for a control reagent was accomplished by precipitation with human IgG by titrating the antiserum with IgG until a definite antigen (IgG) excess was achieved; the supernatant fluid was then used as a control. Phosphate buffer, 0.01 M., pH 7.4 in 0.15 M sodium chloride, was used for all washes. Specimens were mounted in a fluorescence-free medium (Fluormount).

For each brain section, 0.05 ml of undiluted conjugated antihuman serum (either IgG or albumin) was applied to duplicate sections and incubated for 15, 30, or 60 minutes at 37 C in a moist atmosphere. A third and fourth section from each block was incubated with buffer alone and with unconjugated antiserum, respectively, to evaluate tissue and reagent autofluorescence. A blocking test was performed by preliminary incubation of a fifth section with unconjugated antihuman serum (either IgG or albumin) for 15 minutes at 37 C followed by thorough washing and subsequent incubation with conjugated antiserum. As a further control, an additional section was incubated with conjugated antiserum from which specific antibody was absorbed. Following the incubation, all sections were washed at room temperature in three changes of buffer for five minutes each, dried, mounted, and examined with a fluorescence microscope.

Results

Rough quantitation of intensity and extent of specific fluorescence was attempted by visual inspection (Table). In MS patient BI, seven of seven plaques exhibited specific fluorescence when combined with fluorescein-conjugated anti-IgG. In TU, one of three was positive. In RE, two of two were positive. In each of the remaining four brains, a single plaque was studied and was positive. In most cases, fluorescence in

Histological Activity and Specific IgG Fluorescence of Adjacent 10μ Sections on Old Plaques of Demyelination

Plaques Ranked in Order of Increasing Histological Activity	Immunofluorescent Rating*		
	Plaque Tissue		Surrounding White Matter
	Margin	Central	
None to minimal†			
TU 20‡	0	0	0
TU 19	0	0	0
Minimal to moderate			
BI 21	++	+	+
BU 1	+	+	0
⎰ RE 20	+	+	0
⎱ RE 10	+	+	+
BI 25	++	++	++
TU 6§	++	+	+
BI 1b	+	+	0
BI 27	++	+	+
BI 1a	+	+	+
FL 5	+	++	++
Moderate			
BI 9	+	+	+
SI 4	+	++	+
Moderate to marked			
BI 24	++	+	++

*0=absent; +, present; ++, marked specific IgG fluorescence.

§See Figure.

†All the plaques studied were old. They were subdivided into active and inactive demyelination (minimal, moderate, or marked).[9]

‡Letters represent a patient's coded identification and the number refers to the coronal section from which the specimen was obtained. When individual plaques are bracketed the histological rating was the same.

plaque tissue was located predominantly at the periphery involving the entire circumference (Figure). However, fluorescence was also present in varying degrees in the immediately adjacent white matter and in the vascular and perivascular structures within the plaques. In two plaques studied, central fluorescence was more intense than peripheral.

Comment

By inspection of the data shown in the Table, there appears to be a positive correlation between the activity of the plaque and specific IgG immunofluorescence. Two plaques rated as probably inactive showed no IgG, whereas all the rest of the plaques tested had at least minimal activity and IgG. These results may be of practical importance since an active plaque of demyelination may be detectable by the application of a fluorescein-conjugated antihuman IgG reagent to an unwashed frozen-dried section.

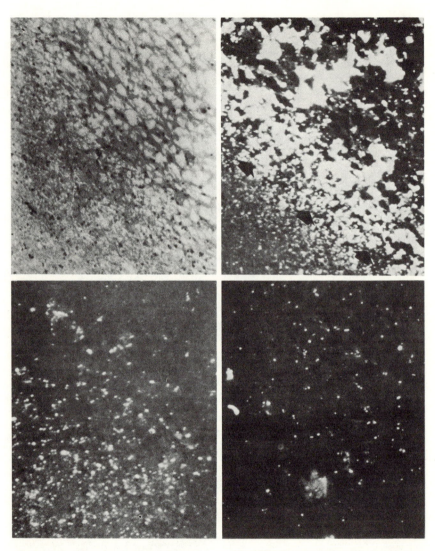

Typical photomicrographs of a plaque of demyelination with surrounding white matter from multiple sclerosis patient BI27 (Table). All photographs are 10μ serial cryostat section, $\times$ 100. **Top left,** Formaldehyde solution fixed and stained with hematoxylin and eosin. The central part of the plaque reveals a relative decrease of cells, numerous astroglial fibers, and enlarged extracellular space (artifact). Mild-moderate hypercellularity can be seen at the plaque margin. The surrounding white matter is probably normal. This old plaque was rated to be moderately active at the margin. **Top right,** Treated with conjugated antihuman IgG reagent. The specific fluorescence was marked at the plaque edge, and present in the normal-appearing white matter **(arrows)**. **Bottom left,** Immunofluorescence control—before the conjugated IgG antibody reagent was applied the tissue was incubated with nonconjugated IgG antibody reagent. Note the extreme reduction of the fluorescence; the little fluorescence seen was primarily autofluorescence, usually orange-tinted rather than green-yellow. **Bottom right,** Immunofluorescence control. The conjugated IgG antibody reagent used had been treated with IgG to absorb the antibodies to IgG. Note the extreme reduction of the fluorescence; the little fluorescence seen was primarily autofluorescence, usually orange-tinted rather than green-yellow.

The terminology proposed by Ibrahim[9] was used in this study. All the microscopic sections taken of the specimens confirmed the gross inspection that each specimen included a plaque of demyelination and white matter surrounding the plaque. The plaques were all of the old type. The histological activity of the plaques was determined without prior knowledge of the immunofluorescence rating. To simplify the grading of the activity of a plaque we relied mainly on one criterion, the degree of cellularity at the plaque margin. It should be noted that the activity of a plaque based on this criterion does not correlate with the intensity of the immunofluorescent stain (Table). For example, BI25 had the most intense specific fluorescence, but was rated seventh out of 15 plaques in degree of histological activity. It is of interest that the plaques with the most intense central fluorescence BI25, FL5 and SI4 had blood vessels in the plaque whose perivascular space was infiltrated by mononuclear cells, very few of which were lipomacrophages. On the other hand, four plaques with 2+ marginal fluorescence and 1+ central fluorescence had no visible associated perivascular cuff in the plaque. Moreover, one of six plaques graded 1+ in the margin and central areas had a blood vessel in the plaque with perivascular cuffing. These observations indicate that plaque margin hypercellularity is sufficient and necessary for the presence of IgG but the presence of perivascular infiltration of mononuclear cells can further add to the concentration. It is possible that a decreased blood-brain barrier would raise the IgG content in the brain; however, this was not considered reasonable in view of the fact that the concentration of albumin, a smaller protein molecule, was not increased, either by chemical methods[5] or by immunofluorescence, as in the present study.

The nine specimens whose white matter surrounding a plaque showed specific IgG fluorescence all had positive plaques. Furthermore, only two had visible abnormalities in the white matter (minimal perivascular cuffing of mononuclear cells, very few of which were lipomacrophages). The finding of specific IgG fluorescence in the white matter immediately adjacent to plaque tissue with elevated IgG concentration (Table and Figure) supports our previous observation that these regions can have a higher IgG concentration than control white matter despite normal histological appearance.[5,7] These observations may support the hypothesis that IgG diffuses into the normal-appearing white matter from an area of disease where cells capable of synthesizing IgG exist.

IgG was not identified by this technique in the disease-control tissues employed, except within blood vessels, in spite of marked alterations in brain structure and extensive tissue damage; this suggests a relatively specific accumulation of IgG in MS tissue. Similarly, albumin was not identified in any except within blood vessels.

Identification of the cells associated with the most intensely stained areas was attempted but was not possible, probably because of technical factors such as the use of postmortem tissue and the artifacts introduced by drying of the tissue sections; however, another possibility has occurred to us. If the majority of the IgG was located in the enlarged extracellular spaces within plaques[10] perhaps its fluorescence overshadowed the intracellular localization. Inspection of the photomicrographs (Figure) suggested that much of the specific fluorescence was in acellular areas as revealed by dark-field illumination. Moreover, with modest washing of the sections (phosphate buffer, formaldehyde solution or acetone) there was a significant reduction of the specific immunofluorescence—this result suggests that the majority of the IgG was unbound or easily extractable; perhaps located extracellularly. Experiments are under way to evaluate the validity of this hypothesis. Therefore, the significant question of the cellular localization of IgG in MS brain tissue is as yet unanswered.

The immunological specificity of these reactions is crucial to their interpretation. These problems have been stressed at length by Coons,[11] Beutner,[12] and Nairn.[13] In control experiments, autofluorescence was minimal and approximately equal in the MS and control tissues after the application of buffer alone and after the application of unconjugated antiglobulin. In the blocking tests, decreased to absent specific staining was consistently found (Figure). As pointed out by Coons and by Nairn, the antigen-antibody complex may be replaced by conjugated antibody during staining; therefore, complete absence of specific fluorescence may not be found. The test is considered valid if a significant decrease of specific staining is produced. Removal of specific antibody from the fluorescein-conjugated antiserum by titration with a specific antigen (IgG) to a point of antigen excess resulted in a reagent exhibiting no specific fluorescence when added to plaque tissue previously noted to have such fluorescence (Figure). Finally, the brain specimens used in these experiments were not perfused before freezing; some serum IgG and albumin remained within the blood vessels and reacted appropriately to the specific reagents and controls. Therefore, these intravascular proteins served to indicate activity of the specific conjugated antisera.

This study was supported by the Horace H. Rackham School of Graduate Studies, University of Michigan (NSF Institutional Grant 98) and Public Health Service grant NB 05388-04.

References

1. Kabat, E.A.; Moore, D.H.; and Landow, H.: An Electrophoretic Study of the Protein Components in the Cerebrospinal Fluid and Their Relationship to Serum Proteins, *J Clin Invest* 21:571 (Sept) 1942.

2. Yahr, M.D.; Goldensohn, E.S.; and Kabat, E.A.: Further Studies on the Gamma Globulin Content of Cerebrospinal Fluid in Multiple Sclerosis and Other Demyelinating Disease, *Ann NY Acad Sci* 58:613 (July 28) 1954.

3. Frick, E., and Scheid-Seydel, L.: Untersuchungen mit J[131]-markiertem gamma-globulin zur Frage der Abstammung der Liquoreiweisskörper, *Klin Wschr* 36:66 (Jan 15), and 857 (Sept 15) 1958.

4. Tourtellotte, W.W., and Parker, J.A.: Multiple Sclerosis: Correlation Between Immunoglobulin-G in Cerebrospinal Fluid and Brain, *Science* 154:1055 (Nov 25) 1966.

5. Tourtellotte, W.W., and Parker, J.A.: Multiple Sclerosis: Brain Immunoglobulin-G and Albumin, *Nature* 214:683 (May 13) 1967.

6. Tourtellotte, W.W., and Parker, J.A.: "Some Spaces and Barriers in Postmortem Multiple Sclerosis," in Lajtha, A., and Ford, D.H. (eds.): *Progress in Brain Research: Brain Barrier Systems,* New York: Elsevier Publishing Co., 1968, vol 29, pp 493-525.

7. Tourtellotte, W.W.; Parker, J.A.; and Itabashi, H.H.: Source of Elevation of Gamma Globulin in Brain Tissue From Patients With Multiple Sclerosis, *Trans Amer Neurol Assoc* 91:351, 1966.

8. Kabat, E.A., and Mayer, M.M.: *Experimental Immunochemistry,* ed 2, Springfield, Ill: Charles C Thomas, Publishers, 1961, p 25.

9. Ibrahim, M.Z.M.: "Histochemistry Applied to Neuropathology," in Adams, C.W.M. (ed.): *Neurochemistry,* Amsterdam: Elsevier Publishing Co., 1965, p 454.

10. Périer, O., and Grégoire, A.: Electron Microscopic Features of Multiple Sclerosis Lesions, *Brain* 88:937 (Dec) 1965.

11. Coons, A.H.: "Fluorescent Antibody Methods," in Danielli, J.F. (ed.): *General Cytochemical Methods I.* New York: Academic Press, Inc., 1958, p 399.

12. Beutner, E.H.: Immunofluorescent Staining: The Fluorescent Antibody Method, *Bact Rev* 25:49 (Jan) 1961.

13. Nairn, R.C.: *Fluorescent Protein Tracing,* Baltimore: Williams & Wilkins Co., 1962, pp 120-121.

Epidemiological Studies

Mortality and migration in multiple sclerosis

John F. Kurtzke, M.D., Leonard T. Kurland, M.D.,

and Irving D. Goldberg, M.P.H.

IN THE EPIDEMIOLOGY of multiple sclerosis (MS), one aspect that has had increasing attention in recent years is the study of migrant populations to or from different risk areas throughout the world. The basic questions are twofold: Does the migrant carry with him the risk of his land of birth? If so, is there a critical age at which this risk is no longer operative?

In the United States the weight of available evidence indicates that the country can be divided into two parts in reference to the risk of MS: a high-risk region north of 37 or 38° north latitude and a lower-risk region south of that line. Prevalence studies from the 1950s suggest a rate of about 50 per 100,000 population in northern United States and southern Canada, with a range of 30 to 60 per 100,000. In southern United States the rates ranged from 5 to 15 and averaged about 10 per 100,000 population, and this area is part of what has been considered a medium-risk area. In Europe a similar division between high- and medium-risk regions seemed to hold for areas north or south, respectively, of about 45° north latitude.

This paper concerns mortality data associated with migration into and within the United States.

METHODS AND MATERIALS

The American Public Health Association undertook an intensive investigation into the cause-of-death data in the United States. A series of monographs has resulted. One of these discusses neurologic and sense organ disorders, and the data that follow were obtained from its chapter on multiple sclerosis.

All deaths in the United States for 1959 through 1961 were ascertained, and those coded to MS (7th ISC[4] code 345) as the primary, or underlying, cause of death were distributed according to state of birth and death and by age, sex, and color. Immigrants were denoted according to place of death and country of origin as well as by age, sex, and color.

Crude average annual death rates per 100,000 population were obtained by summing the deaths for the three years 1959-61 and relating them to three times the 1960 population census for the appropriate age, sex, color, or state. Age-adjusted death rates were similarly calculated, with adjustment by the direct method to the 1940 United States census population.[5]

RESULTS

The 1959-61 average annual crude death rate for MS for all ages combined was 0.8 per 100,000 population. Age-specific death rates by sex and color are shown in Table 1. Rates were negligible for those less than 15 years of age, increased sharply and steadily to a plateau for the group between 45 and 64 years of age, and then declined. Rates for females

TABLE 1

AVERAGE ANNUAL AGE-SPECIFIC MORTALITY RATES PER 100,000 POPULATION FOR
MS ACCORDING TO SEX AND COLOR, UNITED STATES, 1959-61

Age (years)	Total	Total Male	Female	White Total	White Male	Female	Nonwhite Total	Nonwhite Male	Female
Less than 15	0.0*	0.0*	0.0*	0.0*	0.0*	0.0*	0.0*	−†	0.0*
15-24	0.1	0.1	0.1	0.1	0.1	0.1	0.1*	0.0*	0.2*
25-34	0.5	0.4	0.5	0.4	0.3	0.5	0.5	0.6	0.5
35-44	1.2	0.9	1.5	1.3	0.9	1.6	1.0	0.9	1.1
45-54	2.0	1.6	2.2	2.1	1.7	2.3	1.0	0.7	1.3
55-64	2.0	1.9	2.1	2.1	2.0	2.2	1.1	0.9*	1.4
65-74	1.9	2.1	1.8	2.0	2.2	1.9	0.6*	0.7*	0.5*
75-84	1.5	1.7	1.3	1.5	1.8	1.3	0.7*	0.7*	0.8*
85 and older	0.8	1.3*	0.5*	0.9	1.4*	0.6*	−†	−†	−†
All ages	0.8	0.7	0.9	0.8	0.7	0.9	0.4	0.4	0.5

* Rate based on less than 20 deaths in three years
† No deaths in three years

to age 65 exceeded those for males; in general, rates for males at most ages tended to equal those for females who were ten years younger. Rates for nonwhites were based on less than 100 deaths a year for all ages and both sexes combined. From the age of 35 years on, the rates for nonwhites were lower than the rates for whites for almost every age group, regardless of sex.

Age-adjusted death rates by U.S. census region according to sex and color are noted in Table 2. Many of these rates, especially those for nonwhites, are unstable because of the small numbers in specific age classes used in the adjustment method.

Generally, age-adjusted death rates for MS among the white foreign-born population of the United States were somewhat lower than those among the native-born whites: 0.6 and 0.7 for foreign-born males and females, respectively, versus 0.7 and 0.9 for the native Americans. There were, however, notable differences according to country of origin among the foreign-born whites. Table 3 lists the death rates for immigrants from countries that provided more than 5 deaths due to MS in the three years 1959-61 *and* were represented in the international comparisons made by Goldberg

TABLE 2

AVERAGE ANNUAL AGE-ADJUSTED MORTALITY RATES PER 100,000 POPULATION FOR MS BY SEX, COLOR, AND CENSUS REGION, UNITED STATES, 1959-61

Census region	Male	Female	White	Nonwhite
New England	0.9	1.1	1.0	1.0
Middle Atlantic	0.8	1.0	0.9	0.8
East North Central	0.8	1.0	1.0	0.5
West North Central	0.8	1.0	0.9	0.6
South Atlantic	0.5	0.7	0.6	0.5
East South Central	0.4	0.5	0.5	0.5
West South Central	0.4	0.4	0.4	0.4
Mountain	0.8	1.0	0.9	0.2
Pacific	0.7	0.8	0.8	0.2
Total United States	0.7	0.8	0.8	0.5

and Kurland[6] for MS deaths in various countries within the 1950-58 period. The unpublished crude rates for the foreign lands are cited rather than the published age-adjusted rates to provide some comparability with the U.S. death rates among the foreign-born, which are also crude (unadjusted) rates.

The uniformity between the rates for the immigrants and those of their native lands suggests that immigrants, in general, retain the

TABLE 3

AVERAGE ANNUAL CRUDE MS DEATH RATES PER
100,000 POPULATION ACCORDING TO BIRTHPLACES
OF FOREIGN-BORN WHITES WHO DIED IN THE
UNITED STATES, 1959-61, COMPARED WITH
REPORTED RATES FOR NATIVES OF THE SAME
COUNTRIES, 1950-58

Country of origin	Immigrant rates (United States)	Native rates for country of origin
Ireland	2.9	2.8
Germany	1.6	2.3*
Czechoslovakia	1.5†	2.1
Austria	2.3	2.2
Norway	1.7†	1.7
Canada	1.6	1.0
Sweden	1.7†	1.2
Italy	1.0	0.7
Mexico	0.5†	0.1

* West Germany

† Rate based on less than 20 but more than 5 deaths in three years

MS risk of their homeland. However, most of the data concern immigration from one high-risk area to another.[7]

The geographic distribution within the United States for MS death rates according to state of residence at death is shown in Figure 1 for all inhabitants, regardless of origin, sex, or color. Generally, the states located north of 37° north latitude have high rates and those south of this latitude have uniformly low rates. In Figure 2, similar data are drawn for state of birth for all native-born Americans of both sexes and colors combined. The high-rate states are north of 37° north latitude and the low-rate states are south of it. If we limit attention to the whites who died of MS while resident of the same state in which they were born, we see the reasonably consistent division into a high-rate north and a low-rate south by 37° north latitude (Fig. 3). Exceptions in the North are chiefly states with few native deaths.

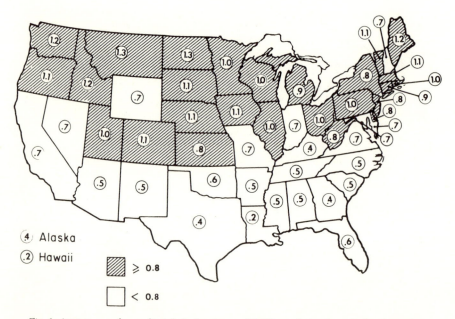

4 Alaska
2 Hawaii

▨ ≥ 0.8
☐ < 0.8

Fig. 1. Average annual age-adjusted death rates per 100,000 population for multiple sclerosis by state, according to residence at death, both sexes, and white and nonwhites, United States, 1959-61

66

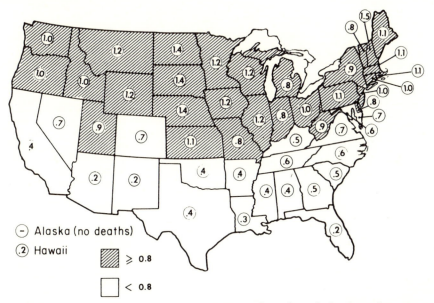

Fig. 2. Average annual crude death rates per 100,000 population for multiple sclerosis by state, according to residence at birth, both sexes, and whites and nonwhites, United States, 1959-61

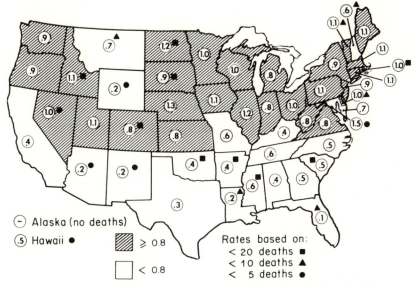

Fig. 3. Average annual crude death rates per 100,000 population for multiple sclerosis by state, whites only, where state of birth and death residence is the same, United States, 1959-61

TABLE 4

DEATHS FROM MS AMONG U.S. NATIVE-BORN BY CENSUS REGIONS
OF BIRTH AND DEATH, 1959-61, AND THREE-YEAR POPULATIONS IN
EACH REGION BY BIRTHPLACE, BASED ON 1960 U.S. CENSUS

Region of death	Region of birth						
	Northern tier				Southern tier		
	North East	Middle Atlantic	East North Central	West North Central	South Atlantic	East South Central	West South Central
Northern tier							
New England							
MS deaths	265	24	3	1	6	0	0
Population (10^3)	23,962	1,725	402	172	556	129	121
Middle Atlantic							
MS deaths	24	738	25	13	36	8	2
Population (10^3)	1,540	77,619	1,585	511	4,372	683	380
East North Central							
MS deaths	5	34	774	45	32	32	5
Population (10^3)	492	3,069	81,382	3,206	3,114	6,234	1,617
West North Central							
MS deaths	3	5	41	356	3	4	7
Population (10^3)	126	403	2,359	37,776	339	705	1,461
Southern tier							
South Atlantic							
MS deaths	14	31	36	4	328	16	4
Population (10^3)	1,035	4,059	2,686	875	60,983	2,953	801
East South Central							
MS deaths	0	1	6	2	7	146	1
Population (10^3)	84	286	857	273	1,292	31,730	689
West South Central							
MS deaths	1	1	7	15	4	17	139
Population (10^3)	166	531	1,097	1,691	792	1,921	41,367

Some measure of migration can be achieved by considering those whose state of birth and state of death differ. It is impossible to determine from death data, however, the age at which such migration took place or the duration or frequency of any such changes. Nor do we know whether or how the disease influenced migration. In this manner also, only that fraction of the actual migrants between states who had different residences at birth and death can be identified, and any state of residency other than those for birth and death is unknown. Further, if a migrant returned to his birthplace before death, he was identified as a "nonmigrant." Still, for those whose residences at birth and death were in different states, this is a valid indication of migration.

To study migration between residence of birth and death from these data, however, we need areas larger than states because the number of such migrants is small. We also need geographic divisions that separate the high-risk northern states from the low-risk southern states. As noted in Table 2, the country has been divided in such a fashion into 9 regions, as established by the Bureau of the Census. The 2 most western regions, Mountain and Pacific, extend from Canada to Mexico and are therefore of no use in this context. However, the eastern two-thirds of the United States is divided into a northern tier of 4 census regions—New England, Middle Atlantic, East North Central, and West North Central—and a southern tier of 3 regions—South Atlantic, East South Central, and West South Central. These tiers are reasonably close to defining the risk areas that we would like to separate.

Table 4 details the number of MS deaths

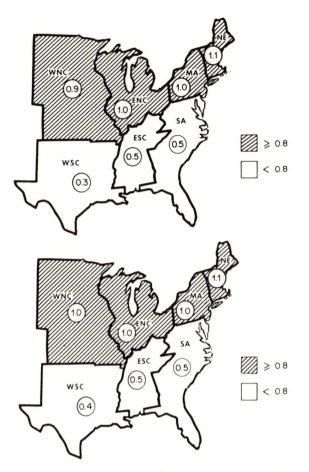

Fig. 4. Average annual crude death rates per 100,000 population for multiple sclerosis within 7 of the 9 census regions, where region of birth and death residence is the same, United States, 1959-61

Fig. 5. Average annual crude death rates per 100,000 population for multiple sclerosis within 7 census regions for those whose residence at birth and death was in the same tier (northern or southern), according to region of death residence, United States, 1959-61

during 1959-61 and the three-year population at risk, according to the 7 census regions of birth and death. The population is for those who resided in the given census region in 1960 but had been born in each individual region as identified. Crude death rates for those whose residence at birth and at death was within the same census region, the major diagonal of Table 4, are drawn in Figure 4. We note the persistence of north high-risk versus south low-risk MS regions.

Figure 5 includes the death rates for those who had migrated *within* their own tier, northern or southern, according to their residence at

death. For example, a rate of 1.1 per 100,000 is cited for New England. This was the result of 293 deaths from MS in New England, which included the 265 born in New England plus the 28 migrants who were born in other northern regions but died while resident in New England: 24 born in Middle Atlantic; 3, in East North Central; and 1, in West North Central. If we exclude those who were born and died in the same region and limit attention only to the "true" migrants from northern regions to other northern regions, then the death rates by place of death were 1.2 for New England, 1.7 for Middle Atlantic, 1.2

69

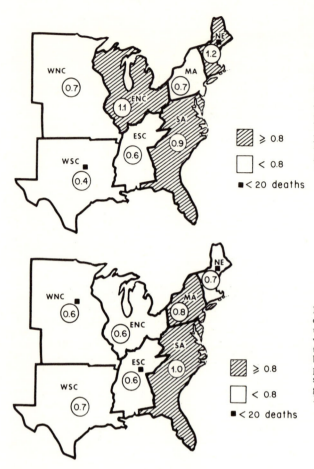

Fig. 6. Average annual crude death rates per 100,000 population for multiple sclerosis within 7 census regions for those whose residence at birth and death was in opposite tiers (northern or southern), according to region of birth, United States, 1959-61

Fig. 7. Average annual crude death rates per 100,000 population for multiple sclerosis within 7 census regions for those whose residence at birth and death was in opposite tiers (northern or southern), according to region of death, United States, 1959-61

for East North Central, and 1.7 for West North Central, or a rate of 1.4 per 100,000 population for all northern migrants within the northern tier.

The southern tier in the same manner showed rates of 0.5 (South Atlantic and East South Central) and 0.4 (West South Central) according to region of death for all whose birth and death residences were in the southern tier. Even after exclusion of those whose southern region of birth and death was the same, the "true" southern migrants within this tier had rates of 0.5 (South Atlantic), 0.4 (East South Central), and 0.8 (West South Central), for a total rate of 0.6 among the southern migrants within the southern tier.

Accordingly then, movement within the tier—northern or southern—preserved the north-south differential in the risk of MS.

Figure 6 lists the MS death rates for those whose death residence was in the tier opposite to that of birth, according to their individual region of birth. For example, the rate of 1.2 for New England was based on 15 persons who had been born in New England but who died of MS in any 1 of the 3 southern regions.

70

The other rates for the northern regions were based on 33, 49, and 21 MS deaths for the Middle Atlantic, East North Central, and West North Central regions of birth, respectively.

The rates for the southern tier were generated from 77 (South Atlantic), 44 (East South Central), and 14 (West South Central) deaths among persons with MS who were born in those regions but died while resident in the northern tier.

Because the combination of regions differs when region of death is specified, we note in Figure 7 the migration patterns with the MS death rates expressed according to region of death residence for those who had been born in the opposite tier. The rate of 0.7 for New England then refers to the 6 persons who had been born in 1 of the 3 southern regions but who died of MS while resident in New England. Numbers underlying the other rates for the northern tier of 0.8, 0.6, and 0.6 were 46, 69, and 14, respectively, from east to west. In the southern tier, the respective numbers of deaths were 85, 9, and 24 for rates of 1.0, 0.6, and 0.7.

Although some of these rates for migrants are based on small numbers, the overall impression remains that changing tiers between birth and death has virtually obliterated the striking north-south difference in risk seen for all MS deaths by place of birth and death *or* for those who had migrated only within the tier. Changing tiers resulted in all the regional death rates coming closer to the MS death rate for the country as a whole. It seemed to matter little as to the direction of change or the time (birth vs. death).

This conclusion is summarized in Table 5. There was a highly significant difference (p <0.0001) between rates for northern and southern tiers for those whose birth and death residences were in the same tier—1.00 northern vs. 0.46 southern. For those who changed tiers of residence between birth and death, the difference is no longer significant (p > 0.05): born in the northern and died in the southern tier was 0.87 and born in the southern and died in the northern tier was 0.68. Additional assessment can be made for these rates. If migration after birth had no effect on MS death rates, then the rates for those who changed tiers should not differ from those who did not

TABLE 5

DEATHS AND DEATH RATES FOR MS AMONG U.S. NATIVE-BORN, 1959-61, ACCORDING TO RESIDENCE AT BIRTH AND DEATH WITHIN THE NORTHERN AND SOUTHERN TIERS

| | Place of birth | |
Place of death	Northern tier	Southern tier
Death rates per 100,000 population ± SD		
Northern tier	1.00 ± 0.02	0.68 ± 0.06
Southern tier	0.87 ± 0.08	0.46 ± 0.02
MS deaths, three-year totals		
Northern tier	2,356	135
Southern tier	118	662
Three-year population from 1960 census*		
Northern tier	236,330,000	19,709,000
Southern tier	13,641,000	142,528,000

* Differences from Table 4 due to rounding

change tiers. The southern-born who died of MS while living in the North did show a significant difference (p <0.001), with a rate of 0.68 versus the southern nonmigrant rate of 0.46. The comparison for the northern-born in this fashion was not statistically significant (p ≅ 0.10); here, the rate was 0.87 for the northern-born who resided and died in the South versus 1.00 for those who were born and resided in the North. On the assumption that the findings are valid, these last analyses would be compatible with the hypothesis that among those who die of MS, residence in the northern tier at some time *after* birth carries a higher risk because the southerners on moving had a significantly higher rate than those remaining in the South, while the northerners who moved south retained some, but not all, of their higher MS risk.

DISCUSSION

Investigation of disease from death-certificate data in this country has long been considered unreliable because of doubts as to the accuracy and the adequacy of such certificates. There is considerable information that those coded to MS as the underlying, or primary, cause of death reflect appreciable errors of commission and omission. Still, the availability of death data for MS provides a broad overview of the disorder, and the data are the only resource currently available for nationwide information on this disease in the United States.

Of course, all epidemiologic inquiries are open to question. Diagnostic variations, input bias, and incomplete ascertainment—all are relevant, whether one is considering a population prevalence study or death-certificate data. Therefore, it is essential to seek support from other approaches for any conclusions or inferences attained in any epidemiologic work. That this is also required a fortiori in hospital case series seems not well recognized by many clinicians.

The mortality data for MS considered herein agree with the many prevalence studies of this disease that indicate the high risk of MS in the northern states and the notably lower risk in the southern states. Evidence for a smooth gradient increasing regularly with latitude seems minimal, and a dichotomous distribution north and south of the 37° parallel of north latitude seems more likely.

The rates for the foreign-born residents of the United States were about the same as the rates for their lands of birth. If valid, this would suggest that immigrants in general carry their risk of MS with them. The death data could be dismissed as a curious coincidence if there was not some support for this hypothesis. Table 6 summarizes this information. To the left are listed sites to which the immigrants came, together with prevalence rates for probable MS among the natives of these sites. They are grouped into low-, medium-, and high-risk areas. To the right are listed the prevalence rates for probable MS among the immigrants to these sites, according to whether their own land of origin is an area of high, medium, or low risk for MS.[7] The high-risk areas are northern United States, Canada, and northern and central Europe. The medium-risk areas refer to southern Europe but also include southern United States and probably Australia. The low-risk areas are Asia and Africa.

From the study of immigrants to Israel by Alter et al.,[8] we have selected the 38 immigrants from Germany, Austria, Hungary, and Czechoslovakia as coming from the high-risk area, the 5 from southern Europe, including Turkey, as coming from the medium-risk area, and the 17 from those regions of Asia and Africa that had defined populations[8] as coming from the low-risk area.

The rates for the Netherlands Antilles as

TABLE 6

PREVALENCE RATES PER 100,000 POPULATION FOR PROBABLE MS AMONG IMMIGRANTS, GROUPED ACCORDING TO MS RISK OF THEIR NATIVE LANDS, COMPARED WITH RATES FOR NATIVES OF THE IMMIGRATION SITE

Immigration site	Rates for native-born of immigration site	MS risk of immigrants' native land		
		High	Medium	Low
To low-risk areas				
Israel[9]	4	33	8	3
Netherlands Antilles[9]	3	59		
Republic of South Africa[10,11]	6	48	15	
Hawaii*[12]	5	— 35 —		
To medium-risk areas				
Queensland[13,14]	9	15		
Western Australia[15]	10	31		
Perth, Western Australia[16,17]	14	22		
Perth, Western Australia[18]	40†	84†		
To higher-risk areas				
Southern Australia*[19]	38	37	4	

* Definition of multiple sclerosis unclear
† Rate for those aged 40 to 49 years only

described by Moffie[9] are based on 5 natives and 9 immigrants, mostly from the Netherlands. In the works of Dean[10] and Kurtzke et al.,[11] immigrants to the Republic of South Africa from northern and central Europe had a rate of 48 per 100,000, based on 114 patients (as revised), while the 4 from southern Europe provided a rate of 15. The native rate of 6 was for 158 white South Africans. In Hawaii, Alter et al.[12] found a prevalence rate of 5 for the 33 native-born Hawaiians. There were 44 immigrants to Hawaii, all white, three-fourths from northern areas of the United States or other such lands of the western hemisphere and half the remainder from "intermediate" areas between 30 and 35° north latitude of the same hemisphere. Alter and his associates' definition of MS was "the Allison criteria" but it is not clear whether this included "possible MS."

Australia seems generally to fall within the medium-risk MS zone. Rates for immigrants to Western Australia have been recalculated for those from Europe alone, and these 23 patients provide a prevalence of 31 per 100,000 in opposition to the rate of 10 for the 68 native-born, as reported by Saint and Sadka.[15] In Perth, Western Australia, McCall et al.[16] and McCall[17] found a rate of 14 for the 44 natives and 22 for the 15 European immigrants. McCall et al.[18] also provided age-specific prevalence rates for those aged 40 to 49 years: the native rate was 40 per 100,000 whereas that for the European immigrants was 84. In Queensland, however, there was little difference between the natives (with a prevalence of 9 from 99 patients) and immigrants from the United Kingdom (with a rate of 15 from 14 patients) according to Sutherland et al.[13,14]

Rischbieth[19] studied the State of South Australia. His definition of MS was not clear and perhaps possible MS was included. His rates for native-born and those for northern European immigrants were virtually the same, 38 for 294 natives and 37 for 30 such immigrants. However, for southern Europe a rate of only 4 per 100,000, based on 1 immigrant, was recorded.

Immigration restrictions in Australia may perhaps have affected the data, but in general one might conclude that the immigrant carries the MS risk of his native land with him.

We then looked for information as to whether there is a critical age at which this carrying of risk is operant. Table 7 summarizes the relevant data from a study of U.S. Army patients with MS in World War II.[20,21] Cited are the ratios of MS cases to matched controls according to residence at different periods. The significant differential in risk between northern and southern tiers, which was noted for residence at birth and at induction, was absent for residence in service but before clinical onset of MS. This probably means that the critical age at acquisition is well before clinical onset. In this study, neither birth nor induction ages could be defined as the critical ones because, for about 85% of the men, places of birth and induction were the same.

Here then is where the mortality data among U.S. migrants previously presented are relevant. It was clear that the north-south differential was present for residence at birth and at death and for those whose birth and death locales were within the same northern or southern tier. However, changing tiers between birth and death virtually destroyed this differential. *If* the critical age for acquisition of MS were at birth or near it, there should have been, for those who changed tiers between birth and death, persistence of the significant differential in risk but with a *reversal* of the MS death rates so that the northern tier would have had the significantly low rates and the southern tier the high rates. This was not found, and indeed the southern-born who died in the North had a death rate significantly higher than the southern nonmigrants; the inference then is that the critical age for the acquisition of MS is well beyond birth.

TABLE 7

RESIDENCE BY TIER IN UNITED STATES AT BIRTH, AT INDUCTION, AND IN SERVICE, EXPRESSED AS CASE-CONTROL RATIOS, FOR MS PATIENTS IN THE ARMY IN WORLD WAR II[20,21]

Tier	Birth	Time of residence Induction	In service*
Northern	1.45	1.38	1.03
Middle	0.86	0.86	0.99
Southern	0.75	0.80	1.07
Total	1.01	1.00	1.03
No. of residences	373	388	578
p	<0.01	<0.01	>0.10

* Residences in service prior to clinical onset only

From the death data we look for an age well after birth and from the Army data for an age well before clinical onset. Acquisition between about age 10 and 15 years was hypothesized on rather fragmentary geographic data[22] and from MS siblings in England who were living together.[23] More recent evidence is available from Israel[24] and South Africa.[11,25] In these studies, the risk of MS for immigrants from Europe was high *only* for those who were more than 15 years old at immigration, and there were few with MS among those who had been less than 15 years old at immigration. In South Africa, the prevalence rate for northern European immigrants less than 15 years old at migration approximated that for the English-speaking native white South Africans, whereas for immigrants older than 15 years upon arrival the rates were similar to those for their native lands. In Hawaii, too, few of the immigrants with MS had entered that land before 15 years of age.[12] In 1961, Wainerdi[26] entitled his paper, "Does the multiple-sclerosis syndrome begin at puberty?" At this date, the answer could well be in the affirmative.

ACKNOWLEDGMENT

The United States mortality data for 1959-61 were prepared for the American Public Health Association with the support of USPHS grant CH00075 from the Division of Community Health Services, Bureau of State Services, United States Public Health Service, Department of Health, Education, and Welfare to serve as the basis for the APHA Monograph Series of the Vital and Health Statistics Program, Carl T. Erhardt, Sc.D., chief editor.

REFERENCES

1. Spiegelman M: The organization of the vital and health statistics monograph program. In: Emerging Techniques in Population Research. Milbank Memorial Fund, 1963, pp 230-249

2. Kurland LT, Kurtzke JF, Goldberg ID: Epidemiology of Neurologic and Sense Organ Disorders (American Public Health Association Monograph). Cambridge, Harvard University Press. In press.

3. Kurtzke JF, Kurland LT, Goldberg ID, et al: Multiple sclerosis. In: Epidemiology of Neurologic and Sense Organ Disorders (American Public Health Association Monograph). Cambridge, Harvard University Press. In press.

4. Manual of the International Statistical Classification of Diseases, Injuries, and Causes of Death. 2 volumes. Geneva, World Health Organization, 1957

5. National Office of Vital Statistics: Vital Statistics Rates in the United States 1900-1940 (Chapter IV). Public Health Service, Federal Security Agency. Washington DC, Government Printing Office, 1947

6. Goldberg ID, Kurland LT. Mortality in 33 countries from diseases of the nervous system. World Neurol 3:444-465, 1962

7. Kurtzke JF: An epidemiologic approach to multiple sclerosis. Arch Neurol (Chicago) 14:213-222, 1966

8. Alter M, Halpern L, Kurland LT, et al: Multiple sclerosis in Israel: Prevalence among immigrants and native inhabitants. Arch Neurol (Chicago) 7:253-263, 1962

9. Moffie D: De geografische verbreiding van multipele sclerose. Nederl T Geneesk 110:1454-1457, 1966

10. Dean G: Annual incidence, prevalence, and mortality of multiple sclerosis in white South-African-born and in white immigrants to South Africa. Brit Med J 2:724-730, 1967

11. Kurtzke JF, Dean G, Botha DPJ: A method for estimating the age at immigration of white immigrants to South Africa, with an example of its importance. S Afr Med J 44:663-669, 1970

12. Alter M, Okihiro M, Rowley W, et al: Multiple sclerosis among Orientals and Caucasians in Hawaii. Read at the meeting of the American Academy of Neurology, May 1970, Miami, Fla

13. Sutherland JM, Tyrer JH, Eadie MJ: The prevalence of multiple sclerosis in Australia. Brain 85:149-164, 1962

14. Sutherland JM, Tyrer JH, Eadie MJ, et al: The prevalence of multiple sclerosis in Queensland, Australia: A field survey. Acta Neurol Scand 42(Suppl 19):57-67, 1966

15. Saint EG, Sadka M: The incidence of multiple sclerosis in Western Australia. Med J Aust 49:249-250, 1962

16. McCall MG, Brereton TL, Dawson A, et al: Frequency of multiple sclerosis in three Australian cities—Perth, Newcastle, and Hobart. J Neurol Neurosurg Psychiat 31:1-9, 1968

17. McCall MG: Personal communication, July 12, 1968.

18. McCall MG, Sutherland JM, Acheson ED: The frequency of multiple sclerosis in Western Australia. Acta Neurol Scand 45:151-165, 1969

19. Rischbieth RH: The prevalence of disseminated sclerosis in South Australia. Med J Aust 1:774-776, 1966

20. Beebe GW, Kurtzke JF, Kurland LT, et al: Studies on the natural history of multiple sclerosis. 3. Epidemiologic analysis of the Army experience in World War II. Neurology (Minneap) 17:1-17, 1967

21. Kurtzke JF: Some epidemiologic features compatible with an infectious origin for multiple sclerosis. In: Pathogenesis and Etiology of Demyelinating Diseases. Basel, S Karger AG, 1969, pp 59-81

22. Kurtzke JF: On the time of onset in multiple sclerosis. Acta Neurol Scand 41:140-158, 1965

23. Schapira K, Poskanzer DC, Miller H: Familial and conjugal multiple sclerosis. Brain 86:315-332, 1963

24. Alter M, Leibowitz U, Speer J: Risk of multiple sclerosis related to age at immigration to Israel. Arch Neurol (Chicago) 15:234-237, 1966

25. Dean G, Kurtzke JF: A critical age for the acquisition of multiple sclerosis. Trans Amer Neurol Ass 95:232-233, 1970

26. Wainerdi HR: Does the multiple-sclerosis syndrome begin at puberty? Boston Med Quart 12:44-47, 1961

MULTIPLE SCLEROSIS IN MIGRANTS TO SOUTH AFRICA

GEOFFREY DEAN

From a nationwide study of multiple sclerosis (MS) in the Republic of South Africa, it was determined that the prevalence of MS in 1960 was 3/100.000 population among Afrikaans-speaking and 11/100,000 among English-speaking white South Africans, but was about 50/100.000 for immigrants to the Republic from Northern Europe (including the United Kingdom).

The risk of developing MS among immigrants who came to South Africa from Northern Europe after the age of 15 years was four times greater than among those who immigrated before this age. A comparison was made with the previous risk of developing paralytic poliomyelitis which was also greater among the immigrants than among the white South African born. The epidemiological evidence in South Africa and elsewhere, particularly in Israel, shows that MS is a disease of the environment. The evidence suggests that it is a normal "infection" of childhood in areas of poor hygiene. In areas of good hygiene there may be a delay before the infection takes place with an increased risk of the development of a precarious balance between "allergy" and immunity to the agent, resulting in the syndrome we know as multiple sclerosis.

Studies on the Natural History of

Multiple Sclerosis

John F. Kurtzke, MD,
Gilbert W. Beebe, PhD,
Benedict Nagler, MD,
M. Dean Nefzger, PhD.
Thomas L. Auth, MD,
Leonard T. Kurland, MD,

Estimates of longevity after onset or diagnosis of multiple sclerosis (MS) have been highly variable, and few have been based on data arising out of a numerically large series collected near onset and followed for a lengthy period. Recent evidence has called into question the common concept that MS is generally progressive and usually fatal within five to 20 years.

The US veteran population is an exceptional resource for the study of disease. It comprises an enumerable population, well-indexed at many points of medical interest, and with a potential for long-term follow-up study that is unparalleled in the United States. During World War II a large proportion of the entire population of young men served in the Armed Forces, where medical care was available without regard to prior residence or socioeconomic status. Veterans with service-connected disabilities have been eligible for later medical care under the auspices of the Veterans Administration (VA) again without regard to residence or economic status.

For the study of MS, the veteran population has additional advantages. This diagnosis made one ineligible for military service, so that cases discovered in service should be at or near clinical onset. Furthermore, whenever the diagnosis of MS was entertained in service, neurologic evaluation was unusually thorough as MS was also grounds for medical discharge. For these reasons we selected the World War II Army series for an extensive study[1-4] of the natural history of MS.

The present report is concerned with survival to Jan 1, 1963, with particular attention to the influence of our diagnostic review of cases, and of age at onset and diagnosis, upon the estimates of mortality over time. Other influences on survival will be considered in a later paper.

Materials and Methods

The origin of the series, derivation of the study sample, and the diagnostic reviews, have been previously described.[1] The initial series of 762 cases consists of all identifiable men with 90 or more days of service who received a final diagnosis of MS in an Army hospital during 1942 to 1951.

Final study diagnoses for the 762 men in the series were established by our review of the clinical records. Two diagnostic reviews were made, and both involved independent appraisals of each case by at least three neurologists (B.N., J.F.K., L.T.K., and T.L.A.) using essentially the diagnostic criteria of the Schumacher Committee[5] for "definite" MS. In the first review, only the original World War II Army hospital record was made available. This was done in an attempt to judge the adequacy of diagnosis free from the influence of later events. Realization that there was indeed later information perhaps led to many more judgments of "possible" MS than would otherwise have been warranted. A final decision was made in the second review wherein all available clinical information, including the postwar course to 1962, was also provided, as well as all autopsy findings.

The relation between the two review judgments is shown in Table 1. "Strong possible" cases generally met the requirement of anatomic dissemination, but not the criterion of at least two distinct episodes, or progression, required by the Schumacher Committee.[5] In the reports on the onset bout[4] and the diagnostic bout (unpublished data), the 476 definite and 51 strong possible cases have been combined as the MS series. In this paper we shall call the strong possible MS "probable" MS. The 476 cases of definite MS at final review include 174 not so classed in the first, and we shall consider whether the latter differ appreciably as to mortality from those characterized as definite MS when only the World War II Army hospital records were reviewed.

Mortality, both fact and cause, was ascertained through 1962 by means of VA resources, which have been shown to be 98% complete for World War II veterans generally,[6] and must be assumed to be even more complete for a series such as this, essentially all of whom were rated "eligible" for compensation for service-connected disability.

Cause of death was based upon autopsy records (74 cases), clinical records, and death certificates. Two-thirds of all deaths among the definite MS cases were reviewed by one of us (J.F.K.), and the cause assigned on the basis of all available documentation. Their distribution as to cause was about the same as in the one third not reviewed in detail. Of the 121 deaths among the definite MS cases, 93 were attributed to MS; in 32 there were complete autopsy reports with verification of MS. Since the death information was available to the reviewers at the diagnostic review, these deaths provide no evidence as to the validity of the final clinical diagnoses.

Among the 527 definite and probable MS cases, 293 had had an onset bout *before* the Army diagnostic bout, and for 234 the onset and the diagnostic bout in the Army were the same.[4] The former is called *onset group 1*; the latter, *onset group 2*. Among the 476 definite MS, there were 284 in group 1 and 192 in group 2. Age at onset for the 527 cases is described in Table 2, that for the 476 being essentially the same.

The several portions of the Army World War II experience that can be used to estimate the survival of patients with MS are: (1) the entire series of 762 cases diagnosed by Army physicians in World War II; (2) the 527 we reclassified as definite or probable MS; and (3) the 476 definite MS which met all the criteria of the Schumacher Committee.[5] In addition, the latter two groups can be considered according to the relation between their onset bout and their Army diagnostic bout: group 1, for whom these bouts differ, and group 2, for whom they are the same. Lastly, separate consideration will be paid to the 306 cases we considered to have definite MS in the first review, limited to the Army diagnostic hospitalization.

To describe survival over calendar time one must specify a starting point on the time-scale. The choice is between the dates of onset and of diagnosis, the former being of greater biologic interest, but not always precisely known, and the latter being of less biologic value, but always known. If time from onset is used in a series where observation as to mortality starts only at diagnosis, the only cases that contribute information about survival in the early years are those for whom onset and diagnosis coincide. If such cases are not representative, bias is introduced. If time from diagnosis is used, this source of bias is entirely absent, but it is often difficult then to relate the experience to the natural history of the disease. Here we shall consider survival on both time-scales. Calculation of survival rates is by standard life-table methods.[7] In the calculations from the date of clinical onset, patients are added to the series only as of the date they came under neurologic observation in World War II.

We are interested not only in the probability of survival or death, but also in its dependence upon MS. To measure the impact of a disease, we must use some measure of "normal" survival expected in the absence of the disease in question. One method is to use the appropriate death rates from US vital statistics. Whether US death rates provide valid expectations for veterans may be questioned because all men were medically screened for service. In another study Nefzger[8] calculated the mortality expected when US death rates for 1946 to 1965 were applied to a sample of World War II veterans, and thereby provided age-standardized mortality ratios. In his study, the observed mortality was some 16% below expectation over the 20-

Table 1.—Review Diagnosis on Army Hospital Records of
Diagnostic Bout and on Entire Case Material Accumulated
1959 Through 1962

Group No.	Final Review Diagnosis, Entire Case Material	Review Diagnosis* Based on Army Record of Diagnostic Bout					
		1	2	3	4	5	Total
1	Definite MS	302	168	1	5	...	476
2A	Strong possible (probable) MS	...	51	...	...	...	51
2B	Poor possible MS	...	45	...	...	...	45
3	Not MS	3	62	30	50	1	146
4	Unknown	1	17	...	23	...	41
5	Primary lateral sclerosis	...	3	...	...	...	3
	Total	306	346	31	78	1	762

* The diagnostic categories 1 to 5 are those of the final review diagnosis, except that group 2 was not subdivided in the first review.

year period. For this reason, we have also estimated the mortality to be expected in the present MS series by restricting attention to those deaths that were attributed to causes other than MS. Although we then speak from the specific experience at hand, there are questions as to the validity of this method also. It assumes not only that all deaths are correctly labeled as to cause and that none attributed to MS would have occurred without this disease, but also that the presence of MS makes no more nor less likely death from some other condition, ordinarily considered independent of MS and not a complication or consequence of MS.

Results

Survival in Definite MS Cases.—Greatest clinical interest attaches to the fate of the 476 men who had fulfilled all diagnostic criteria for definite MS.[5] Figure 1 gives the annual survival percentages by onset group, the 284 with an onset bout before the diag-

nostic bout in the Army (group 1), and the 192 (group 2) in whom the Army diagnostic bout was the onset. The scale is broken at 60% survival as a convenience in plotting. The small differences between the two onset groups are within the range of chance, even at ten years after onset. Ninety-five percent confidence intervals on the survival percentages after 23 years are 64% to 76% (group 1), 57% to 80% (group 2), and 64% to 74% (total series). The confidence intervals for group 1 after 25 years are 61% to 74%, and 58% to 73% after 30 years.

Thus, after 20 years of illness, three fourths of the patients are still alive; and about two thirds have survived 25 years and even (with somewhat less assurance) 30 years of disease. The median survival (the point at which one half the original series will be dead) has not yet been determined, and is likely to be beyond 30 years, perhaps 35 years or so, after onset among these young male subjects.

Age	Group 1	Group 2	Total
5-9	0.7	...	0.4
10-14	4.8	0.4	2.8
15-19	17.4	9.0	13.7
20-24	37.5	27.4	33.0
25-29	21.8	29.1	25.0
30-34	11.6	25.6	17.8
35-39	4.8	7.3	5.9
40-44	1.4	1.3	1.3
Total	100.0	100.1	99.9
No.	293	234	527
Mean age	23.8 yr	26.9 yr	25.2 yr

Table 3.—Percentage of Survivors by Years
After Onset of Disease, and by
Final Review Diagnosis

Years After Onset	Definite MS	Definite and Probable MS	Not MS	Total Series
0	100.0	100.0	100.0	100.0
5	96.4	96.9	96.1	95.8
10	90.3	91.4	92.7	91.2
15	82.7	84.5	87.5	84.9
20	73.4	75.8	83.2	78.1
25*	66.1	68.8	(78.6)	72.1
30*	(64.2)	(67.0)	(68.0)	(66.8)
No.	476	527	146	762

* Percentages in parentheses are unstable because of small numbers.

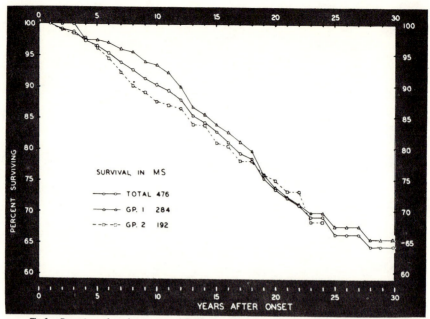

Fig 1.—Percentage of survivors among definite MS cases, by onset group, and by years after onset.

The mortality experience in the 527 definite and probable MS cases is very little different from that in the 476 definite MS cases. For example, at the end of 20 years, survivors represent 73% of the definite MS cases vs 76% of the definite plus probable cases. For both onset groups the difference is also small.

Survival in Relation to Material Used in Diagnostic Review.—The 306 cases classed as definite MS from the clinical records created during the Army diagnostic bout were compared with the 476 similarly designated in our review of the total case. Twenty years after onset, the survival percentages are 70.4% for the 306 cases and 73.4% for the 476 cases, and do not differ significantly. Any bias introduced by the retrospective nature of our review process is therefore small, and we need not hesitate to use the larger series emanating from the final review process.

Survival in Relation to Final Review Diagnosis.—The total series of 762 cases includes 476 definite MS, 527 definite and probable MS, and 146 not-MS cases, as its

major divisions. Survival in these several categories is summarized in Table 3. The not-MS cases suffered from a heterogeneous group of disorders,[1] and it appears fortuitous that their early survival follows so closely that of the MS groups. Certainly, in epidemiologic features, this group differs markedly from the MS.[3]

Survival Dated From Onset or Diagnosis. —The relation between the two time-scales, years from onset and years from diagnosis, is exemplified by Table 4, which also contains survival data for group 1 and group 2 cases by years from diagnosis. Since the two scales are equivalent for the 234 group 2 cases, and for the remaining 293 cases, the median interval from onset to diagnosis is only 39 months,[4] it is not surprising that the two sets of figures for the entire series of 527 men are so similar. Of perhaps greater interest is the comparison of survival for the early onset (group 1) and late onset (group 2) groups, when measured from diagnosis. The difference 20 years after diagnosis is about what one would expect from the three-year difference in median time of on-

Table 4.—Percentage Survival by Years After Diagnosis and After Onset for 527 Definite Plus Probable MS Cases

Years After Onset or Diagnosis	Years Counted From Army Diagnosis			Years Counted From Onset Total Series
	Group 1	Group 2	Total	
0	100.0	100.0	100.0	100.0
5	96.2	97.0	96.6	96.9
10	89.4	90.2	89.8	91.4
15	81.7	83.5	82.5	84.5
20	72.6	78.5	75.1	75.8
No.	293	234	527	527

Table 5.—Percentage Survival After Onset of Definite or Probable MS, by Age at Onset

Years After Onset	Age at Onset					
	15-19	20-24	25-29	30-34	35-39	All Ages
0	100.0	100.0	100.0	100.0	100.0	100.0
5	89.3	97.0	98.9	97.4	96.4	96.9
10	85.7	90.6	93.0	93.0	89.5	91.4
15	82.6	83.5	85.3	85.3	79.8	84.5
20	72.9	75.1	73.8	81.5	72.2	75.8
No.	72	174	132	94	31	527

Table 6.—Observed and Expected* Deaths From All Causes, by Age at Diagnosis, and by Years After Army Diagnosis in 1942 to 1946, Definite and Probable MS Cases Only

Age at Diagnosis	Deaths per 100 Subjects			Percentage Mortality Deficit†	
	Observed	Expected			
		I	II	I	II
Five years after diagnosis					
20-24	3.25	1.06	0	2.2	3.2
25-29	2.13	1.06	0	1.1	2.1
30-34	3.67	1.38	0.93	2.3	2.8
35-39	6.00	2.00	2.04	4.1	4.0
Average	3.31	1.25	0.48	2.1	2.8
Ten years after diagnosis					
20-24	8.13	2.03	1.71	6.2	6.5
25-29	10.64	2.13	0	8.7	10.6
30-34	11.01	3.12	3.88	8.1	7.4
35-39	10.00	5.00	4.17	5.3	6.1
Average	9.93	2.70	2.00	7.4	8.1
Fifteen years after diagnosis					
20-24	13.01	3.01	2.59	10.3	10.7
25-29	15.60	3.83	0	12.2	15.6
30-34	22.94	5.69	7.94	18.3	16.3
35-39	18.00	9.20	8.63	9.7	10.3
Average	17.02	4.70	3.85	12.9	13.7

* Method I uses age-specific and year-specific death rates for US white men; method II, the experience of the MS sample itself after MS deaths were removed by life-table methods.

† The "percentage mortality deficit" at a specific point of observation is obtained as:

$$100 \times \frac{\text{Observed} - \text{expected deaths from 0 to that point}}{\text{Expected survivors at that point}}.$$

set. Although group 1 and group 2 appeared to differ at the time of their onset bout,[4] the suggestion here is that thereafter they may have become quite similar.

Survival According to Age at Onset and at Army Diagnosis.—The influence of age at onset on subsequent survival could be somewhat obscured by factors associated with military selection. Whether a young individual with onset at an early age would pass through the medical screen at induction might well depend on the rate at which his symptoms had progressed, their severity, and residua. In contrast, any major symptoms occurring for the first time in a man already in service would come to medical attention. Thus, there are complex interactions among age at onset, age at diagnosis, and duration of disease at the time observation for mortality begins in this series. That these factors are probably not an important source of bias is suggested by the fact that MS is rarely diagnosed before the age of 18, at which age men became eligible for induction in World War II.

An abstract of the life tables for age-at-onset cohorts is given in Table 5. Although the sampling uncertainties are rather large at both ends of the age range, and one should keep in mind the selective factors mentioned, there is no evidence in this series that age at onset is having any appreciable effect on survival during the first 20 years of follow-up study.

The effect of age is examined more rigorously in Table 6 where each age-at-diagnosis group is first compared with US white men of the same age as to expected survival on a calendar-time scale (method I). The mortality used in calculating these expected values are both age-specific (five-year), and calendar-time-specific (one-year). Calculations were made separately for each year of diagnosis, 1942 to 1946, and summed. In method II, mortality in the MS series itself is used as the basis of expectation, with the 93 deaths from MS treated by life-table methods as losses from observation. Although the agreement between expectations calculated by method I and II is much better than anticipated, in another application, this method might fail utterly, as noted by Ragnar Müller.[9] The agreement does, however, suggest that interaction between

MS and other causes of death was probably not very extensive in this series.

Mortality Deficit Attributable to MS.—From Table 6, the mortality deficit attributable to the disease is about 2% of expected survivors five years after diagnosis, 7% 10 years after, and 13% 15 years after; by the end of 20 years the deficit had risen to 19%. The age cohorts are small and sampling variation is large, but the data contain no suggestion that the percentage mortality deficit is very sensitive to age at diagnosis.

Parallel computations have been made by method II for the 476 definite MS cases, with time counted from onset, and for all ages combined. Table 7 contains a summary of these calculations expressed in terms of relative survival percentages, ie:

$$100 \times \frac{\text{Observed survival percentage}}{\text{Normal survival percentage}}$$

which is equivalent to 100 less the percentage mortality deficit as used in Table 6. The relative survival percentages of Table 7 are numerically very close to the complementary measures in Table 6 for men aged 20 to 39 at diagnosis. Thus, ten years after onset, survival is only 92% of expectation, signifying that 8% of the MS series who, apart from their MS, would have been expected to be alive after ten years have died. Since normal mortality after ten years is only about 2%, this means that about 10% of the MS patients have died, ie, five times normal expectation. The deficit increases rapidly thereafter, from 8% at 10 years, to 21% at 20 years after onset. After 20 years, the normal mortality is about 7% in comparison with 27% observed; conversely, survival 20 years after onset is 79% of normal expectation. This experience is depicted in Fig 2 for the total series, in terms of the normally expected and actually observed survival curves. The shaded portion, the difference between the two curves, provides an estimate of the deficit attributable to the disease. These deficits, divided by the corresponding values on the curve for normal survival, are the complements of the relative survival percentages that appear in Table 7 and are repeated at the bottom of Fig 2. Since the 100% line is an appropriate base line for comparing observed and expected mortality, the vertical scale is broken to permit enlargement of the scale.

Table 7.—Survival in Definite MS Series as Percentage of Normal Survival, by Onset Group

Years After Onset	Percentage of Normal* Survival		
	Group 1	Group 2	Total
0	100	100	100
5	98	97	97
10	95	90	92
15	87	85	86
20	79	81	79
No.	284	192	476

*Normal survival calculated from the non-MS deaths in each onset group (method II).

Table 8.—Terminal Episode in 93 Deaths Attributed to MS

Terminal Episode	No. of Deaths	Subtotal
Pneumonia*	29	
Pneumonia* with cystopyelitis†	30	
Both above with status epilepticus	1	62
Pneumonia* with cardiac failure	2	
Pulmonary embolus and acute exacerbation	3	
Respiratory failure and acute exacerbation	3	7
"Medullary paralysis" (chronic)	1	
Cystopyelitis†	6	
Cystopyelitis† with cardiac failure	2	12
Cardiac failure and/or coronary heart disease	4	
MS (no further data)	12	12
Total		93

* Includes bronchopneumonia, lobar pneumonia, pneumonia unspecified, empyema (one case), and bronchitis (one case) with or without anemia, inanition, or cachexia.
† With or without uremia.

Fig 2.—Estimated mortality deficit attributed to MS, definite cases only, by years after onset.

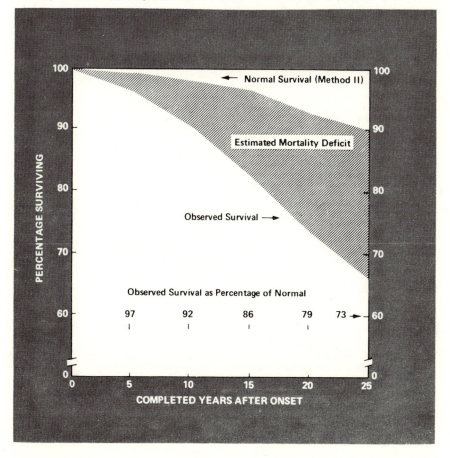

83

Cause of Death.—In the entire Army series of 762 men, there were 162 deaths. In the 51 probable MS cases there was but one death, caused by rheumatic heart disease. Of the 121 deaths among the 476 definite MS cases, 93 were attributed to MS, 24 to unrelated entities, and in 4 cases information was inadequate for judgment. The terminal episode among the 93 with MS as cause of death is detailed in Table 8. Two thirds of the deaths were associated with pneumonitis as a consequence of advanced MS and the bedridden state, and most of the others with sequelae of the neurogenic bladder. Of interest are the acute deaths with pulmonary involvement—three clearly associated with respiratory (ventilatory) failure.

The four "unknown" deaths in the definite MS group involved bronchopneumonia in one, "cerebral hemorrhage due to interstitial nephritis due to MS" in another, and in two there was no information. The relationship of these deaths to MS could not be ascertained as clinical information on recent neurologic dysfunction was unavailable.

The causes of unrelated deaths among the 24 definite MS cases are summarized below:

Trauma	8
Suicide	1
Malignant neoplasm	2
Coronary heart disease	3
Cerebral hemorrhage	1
Postoperative cerebral hemorrhage	1
Perforated peptic ulcer	1
Appendicitis	1
Cirrhosis	2
Alcoholism	1
Addison's disease	1
Erythema multiforme	1
Viral meningoencephalitis	1
Total	24

They are generally what one might expect in a group of young men, with a preponderance of trauma. Only one suicide is recorded in this group.

Among the 44 men whose final review diagnosis was "unknown MS," there were 11 deaths attributed to various causes: malignant brain tumor, luetic heart disease, trauma (two cases), acute cyanide poisoning, suicide, coronary occlusion with myocardial infarction, "bilateral sclerosis" (sic), and unknown cause (three cases).

The group we had classed as "not-MS" on review comprised 146 of the original 762 Army cases. Of these, 27 had died and 17 had been autopsied. Cause of death (which in 12 was the underlying disease which had been mislabeled "MS") for these men is given below:

Where death was due to the underlying neurologic disease:

Brain tumor	7
Basilar aneurysm	1
Syringomyelia	1
Olivopontocerebellar degeneration	1
Dorsolateral sclerosis	1
Myelopathic muscular atrophy	1
Total	12

Where death was unrelated to neurologic disease:

Pulmonary tuberculosis	2
Coronary heart disease	4
Other cardiac disease	2
Cirrhosis	2
Homicide	2
Pulmonary embolus, thrombophlebitis	1
Gastrointestinal hemorrhage, pancreatic calculus	1
Perirenal hemorrhage	1
Total	15

Overall then, deaths from entities unrelated to neurologic disease occurred in about 5% of the 527 MS cases and 10% of the 146 not-MS cases.

Comment

The average duration of any incurable disease is measured by retrospective calculation for patients known to have died of the disease, by prospective study of patients with the disease up to the point when one half of the subjects have died, by following until death all patients known to have the disease and averaging their years of life after onset, or by reconstructing a cohort from the ascertainment of living and deceased cases during a prevalence survey. Retrospective estimation is hazardous and unreliable in the absence of some guarantee that incidence, and the sampling ratio, remained unchanged over the calendar period of estimation. If the series is increasing in size, then it will be biased toward early deaths, for example.

Early reports,[9-15] especially those based on deaths in ordinary clinical series, generally provide estimates of ten years or so, while more recent reports[16-18] give somewhat higher estimates. But there are exceptions. Allison's 1950 estimate of 20 years[11] is one; this was a prospective study wherein he recorded duration from a small series he had personally examined 20 years previously. The next longest duration cited is that of Ipsen[14] obtained by life-table analysis of some 800 MS cases in the Boston area. Ipsen's series is from a period prevalence study of MS, and is actually based on retrospect historical data for those who died during the period of study, 1939 to 1948. Therefore, except for the more sophisticated methodology this work would seem to differ little from the others cited, such as those of Georgi et al[16] or Sällström[15] which too arose from prevalence studies. The grave prognosis for survival in young men suggested by Ipsen[14] in the Boston survey is not confirmed by our material. Although his series was large and carefully analyzed, it would appear to have been biased for men with onset in early adult life.

The average duration of MS calculated from those who have died at a given point in time may be an underestimate for the reasons already cited. The duration in those who have thus far survived is similarly unreliable. Representative figures are provided by Allison[11] at 28 years, Bramwell[12] at 14 years, McAlpine[19] at 18 years, and Percy et al[20] at over 25 years. The limiting factor in Allison's[11] series and in Percy's prospective study,[20] is the small number of cases. Taking into account both those who have died and those still alive, recent authorities generally estimate the average duration of MS to be in excess of 20 or 25 years. Beringer's 1941 estimate[21] of ten years was typical of the era before World War II, and was for the most part based on hospital experience or deaths. Limburg[22] in 1950 had estimated an average duration of some 27 years by subtracting the median age at death from MS according to US mortality statistics from the median age at onset in a number of clinical series. Mackay,[23] Hyllested,[24] and Poeck and Markus[18] are all on record with estimates in excess of 20 years. In their recent review of the subject, McAlpine et al[25] state that average duration should be 25 years or more.

Hyllested's 1961 series[24] was a large one, with 854 deaths (31%) over a ten-year period, but his report does not provide the detail needed to estimate survival in life-table fashion from either onset or diagnosis. MacLean and Berkson's report[26] on 406 essentially nonresident Mayo Clinic cases diagnosed in 1934 to 1939, and followed to 1950, permits a comparison with the present series in terms of years following diagnosis (Table 9). However, the interval between onset and diagnosis was estimated at 7.0 years for the Mayo Clinic series, in comparison with less than two years in the present series. The difference between the foregoing estimates of 79.5% (Mayo) and 89.8% (Army) ten years after diagnosis is equal to a difference of about six to seven years on the curve for the Army series; the two series are probably quite similar.

A small series consisting of all the resident cases of MS from Rochester, Minn has been presented by Percy et al.[20] The experience of this population sample, followed for a lengthy period, may be compared with ours in terms of survival after onset (Table 10). Percy et al[20] also calculated survival as a percent of the normal, using appropriate US mortality statistics for age and sex. Comparison with the definite MS in the Army experience also shows the two series to be very similar (Table 11).

The age distribution of the Army series is not wide enough to represent adequately those whose onset occurs in middle life, when it is generally believed that progressive bouts are more common and prognosis worse. But our study contains no evidence that age at onset or diagnosis is a factor, especially when adjusted for the different levels of mortality normally characteristic of different age groups. The exclusion of women limits the scope of generalization, but for young men it does appear that the present series is a reliable guide to survival. On the basis of the 527 definite and probable cases the calculated survival percentages, and 95% confidence intervals are summarized in Table 12.

Extrapolation of the curve suggests that 50% survival in this series of young men would occur between 30 and 35 years following diagnosis, and about 35 years after onset. The close accord with both Mayo Clinic

Table 9.—Comparison of Survival Rates From Mayo Clinic Nonresident MS Cases and From Present Series, by Years Following Diagnosis

Years After Diagnosis	Mayo Clinic (No. = 406)	Army World War II (No. = 527)
2	97.5	99.6
5	92.7	96.6
10	79.5	89.8

Table 10.—Comparison of Survival Rates From Mayo Clinic Resident MS Cases and From Present Series by Years After Onset

	Percentage Surviving	
Completed Years After Onset	Mayo Resident Series (No. = 46)	Army Series (No. = 527)
5	98	97
10	95	91
15	89	84
20	73	76
25	64	69

Table 11.—Comparison of Survival as Percentages of Normal Survival by Years After Onset for Mayo Clinic Resident MS and for Present Series

	Percentage of Normal Survival	
Completed Years After Onset	Mayo Resident Series (No. = 46)	Army Definite MS (No. = 476)
5	99	97
10	98	92
15	94	86
20	80	79

Table 12.—Percentage Survival Rates With 95% Confidence Intervals for 527 Definite and Probable MS Cases According to Years After Onset

	Percentage Surviving	
Years After Onset	Average	95% Confidence Interval
5	96.9	95-99
10	91.4	89-94
15	84.5	81-88
20	75.8	72-80
25	68.8	63-74

series would suggest that sex is not in fact a major factor in survival, and the contentions of Leibowitz and Alter[27] that young men fare best, and of Ipsen[14] that they do poorly, is not borne out by our experience.

We may predict then that the average duration of life after the onset of MS in young men should be in the order of 35 years or so—a much more optimistic outlook than has generally been taught. The *quality* of survival and predictive features for survival will be topics of later communications.

Summary

In a review of original and follow-up medical records of 762 men given a diagnosis of multiple sclerosis (MS) in Army hospitals during World War II, 476 were judged to have definite MS, 51 "probable MS," 146 "not-MS," and 45 "poor possible" MS, 41 no certain diagnosis, and 3 primary lateral sclerosis. All 762 men have been traced as to survival and cause of death through 1962, and all available clinical and autopsy records critically reviewed. Calculated by life-table methods, survival in the 527 definite and probable MS cases is 76% 20 years after onset, and 69% 25 years after onset.

The indication is that one half of the 527 MS cases, whose average age at onset was 25, will live some 35 years following onset. For the 476 definite MS cases, values are essentially the same: 66% were alive 25 years after onset. The observed mortality of 25% in the MS cases (regardless whether the 476 or the 527 are considered) 20 years after diagnosis is more than three times normal expectation and represents a loss of about 20% of those expected to be alive in a similar group of men subject only to the normal risk of mortality for 20 years. Expressed differently, the MS patients experienced about four fifths of normal survival after 20 years of illness, and about three fourths of normal after 25 years. In the MS series causes of death not attributable to the disease occurred in accord with general expectations as to type and frequency. The major terminal cause when MS was the underlying disease was bronchopneumonia. The overall estimates of survival in this series are little affected by age at onset or diagnosis, the retrospective review procedure, and whether the onset bout preceded the Army diagnostic bout. These findings are in reasonable agreement with several recent studies and estimates as to survival in MS.

This investigation was supported by contract VAm-22734 from the US Veterans Administration, Washington, DC, and is part of a program of medical follow-up studies organized by the NAS-NRC at the request of the Veterans Administration, the Department of Defense, and the Public Health Service.

Funds for supplementary follow-up examinations were provided by the National Multiple Sclerosis Society.

The Medical Statistics Agency, Office of the Surgecn General, Department of the Army, provided the roster of Army personnel with diagnoses of multiple sclerosis during service; records officials in the Veterans Administration and the General Services Administration provided essential records services.

Mrs. Dorothy Mahon and Mrs. Vivian A. Farley of the Follow-up Agency staff gave technical assistance.

References

1. Nagler B, Beebe GW, Kurtzke JF, et al: Studies on the natural history of multiple sclerosis: I. Design and diagnosis. *Acta Neurol Scand* 42(suppl 19):141-156, 1966.

2. Kurland LT, Beebe GW, Kurtzke JF, et al: Studies on the natural history of multiple sclerosis: II. The progression of optic neuritis to multiple sclerosis. *Acta Neurol Scand* 42(suppl 19):157-176, 1966.

3. Beebe GW, Kurtzke JF, Kurland LT, et al: Studies on the natural history of multiple sclerosis: III. Epidemiologic analysis of the army experience in World War II. *Neurology* 17:1-17, 1967.

4. Kurtzke JF, Beebe GW, Nagler B, et al: Studies on the natural history of multiple sclerosis: IV. Clinical features of the onset bout. *Acta Neurol Scand* 44:467-494, 1968.

5. Schumacher GA, Beebe GW, Kibler RF, et al: Problems of experimental trials of therapy in multiple sclerosis: Report by the panel on the evaluation of experimental trials of therapy in multiple sclerosis. *Ann NY Acad Sci* 122:552-568, 1965.

6. Beebe GW, Simon AH: Ascertainment of mortality in the U.S. veteran population. *Amer J Epidem* 89:636-643, 1969.

7. Dublin LI, Lotka AJ, Spiegelman M: *Length of Life*. New York, Ronald Press Co, 1949.

8. Nefzger MD: Follow-up studies of World War II and Korean War prisoners: I. Study plan and mortality findings. *Amer J Epidem*, to be published.

9. Müller R: Studies on disseminated sclerosis with special reference to symptomatology, course and prognosis. *Acta Med Scand* 133(suppl 222):1-214, 1949.

10. Abb L, Schaltenbrand G: Statistische Untersuchungen zum Problem der Multiplen Sklerose: Das Krankheitsbild der Multiplen Sklerose. *Deutsch Z Nervenheilk* 174:199-218, 1956.

11. Allison RS: Survival in disseminated sclerosis: A clinical study of a series of cases first seen twenty years ago. *Brain* 73:103-120, 1950.

12. Bramwell B: Clinical studies: XII. The prognosis in disseminated sclerosis; duration in two hundred cases of disseminated sclerosis. *Edinburgh Med J* 18:16-23, 1917.

13. Carter S, Sciarra D, Merritt HH: The course of multiple sclerosis as determined by autopsy proven cases. *Res Nerv Ment Dis Proc* 28:471-511, 1950.

14. Ipsen J Jr: Life expectancy and probable disability in multiple sclerosis. *New Eng J Med* 243:909-913, 1950.

15. Sällström T: Das Vorkommen und die Verbreitung der Multiplen Sklerose in Schweden: Zur Geographischen Pathologie der Multiplen Sklerose. *Acta Med Scand* suppl 137, pp 1-141, 1942.

16. Georgi F, Hall P, Müller HR: Zur Problematik der Multiplen Sklerose: Geomedizinische Studien in der Schweiz und in Ost-Afrika und ihre Bedeutung für Aetiologie und Pathogenese. *Bibl Psychiat Neurol* 114:1-123, 1961.

17. Müller HR: Die Prognose der Multiplen Sklerose. *Deutsch Med Wschr* 86:1800-1808, 1961.

18. Poeck K, Markus P: Giebt es eine Gutartige Verlaufsform der Multiplen Sklerose? *München Med Wschr* 106:2190-2197, 1964.

19. McAlpine D: The benign form of multiple sclerosis: Results of a long-term study. *Brit Med J* 5416:1029-1032, 1964.

20. Percy AK, Kurland LT, Nobrega FT, et al: Multiple sclerosis in Rochester, Minnesota: A 60 year appraisal. *Trans Amer Neurol Assoc* 93:264-265, 1968.

21. Beringer K: Die Prognose der Multiplen Sklerose. *Deutsch Med Wschr* 67:461-463, 1941.

22. Limburg CC: The geographic distribution of multiple sclerosis and its estimated prevalence in the United States. *Res Nerv Ment Dis Proc* 28:15-24, 1950.

23. Mackay RP: Symposium on nervous and mental disease; multiple sclerosis: Its onset and duration; clinical study of 309 private patients. *Med Clin N Amer* 37:511-521, 1953.

24. Hyllested K: Lethality, duration, and mortality of disseminated sclerosis in Denmark. *Acta Psychiat Neurol Scand* 36:553-564, 1961.

25. McAlpine D, Compston ND, Acheson ED: *Multiple Sclerosis: A Reappraisal*. London, E & S Livingston Ltd, 1965.

26. MacLean AR, Berkson J: Mortality and disability in multiple sclerosis: Statistical estimate of prognosis. *JAMA* 146:1367-1369, 1951.

27. Leibowitz U, Alter M: Clinical factors determining prognosis in multiple sclerosis. *Neurology* 18:286-287, 1968.

Some Epidemiologic Features Compatible
with an Infectious Origin for Multiple Sclerosis

J. F. KURTZKE

Epidemiology is the study of disease characteristics within groups rather than in individual patients. It is concerned with the natural history of a disease, and the discovery of features which differentiate the patient from his unaffected peer. As a field it has proved its worth in the history of medicine by providing clues to the etiology of many infectious, toxic, and nutritional disorders. More recent expansion into the question of chronic illness has led to considerable information about various cancers and degenerative diseases. In neurology, most attention has been paid to the epidemiology of multiple sclerosis (MS), and it would seem appropriate at this time to consider one interpretation of the state of the art in this disorder.

One of the first questions to be raised is where does the disease occur, what is its geographic distribution. The best material to answer this in MS comes from prevalence studies. The prevalence of a disease is the rate derived from the number of cases present in a given population at one time, expressed in cases per unit population. Throughout the world there are about 50 well-performed prevalence studies of MS covering the period since 1945. When the rates from these studies for 'probable' or 'definite' MS are plotted against the geographic latitude of the survey site, we can see that the old teaching of a north-south gradient does not really hold well [1, 2]. In Europe, there is a very sharp drop at about 46° N. latitude (fig. 1). Above this line the prevalence of MS is in the range of 30

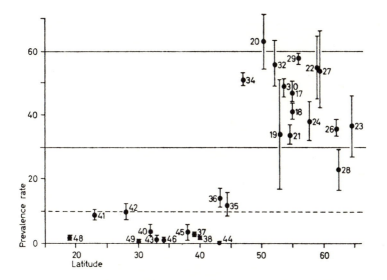

Fig. 1. Prevalence rates for probable MS expressed in cases per 100,000 population correlated with geographic latitude. Dots indicate the rates and the vertical lines the 95 % confidence limits on the rates. Numbers identify the study as in ref. 1: No. 17–36 are from Europe, No. 41, 42 from Australia, No. 37–48 otherwise from Asia, and No. 49 from Africa. Reproduced with permission from Archives of Neurology [2].

to 60 cases per 100,000 population (No. 17–34). In southern Europe (No. 35, 36) rates are near 10 per 100,000, as is also true of Australia (No. 41, 42). In Asia and Africa rates are 0 to 4 per 100,000. Thus we have high, medium, and low frequency zones of MS rather than a smooth rise with latitude.

In the United States and Canada, we see the same high and medium prevalence zones, with the dividing line at about 38° North latitude (fig. 2). The appearance of a gradient here is the result of the study from Washington, D. C. (No. 12) which was limited to hospitalized patients [3]. If, as is generally found, some 70 % of cases in a community will be ascertained from hospital records, one could assign to this city a prevalence rate of about 30 instead of the rate of 21 cited, and therefore this too would be in the high frequency zone of MS. A recent epidemiologic study of MS in US Army men of World War II [4, 5], also points to a sharp division at 38° between two general zones of MS frequency (fig. 3). Here the numbers refer to a ratio of cases to matched controls.

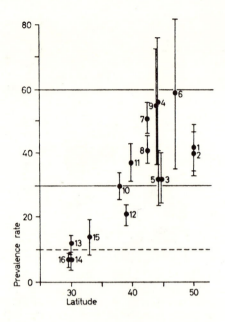

Fig. 2. Prevalence rates for probable MS correlated with latitude, as in figure 1, for Canada (No. 1–5) and United States (No. 6–16). Reproduced with permission from Archives of Neurology [2].

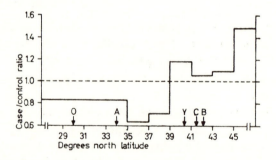

Fig. 3. Residence at birth for MS cases in the US Army during World War II expressed in ratios of cases to matched controls and correlated with geographic latitude. Reproduced with permission from Neurology [4].

When we wish to look more closely at the distribution of MS, we turn to studies wherein one large region was surveyed at one time by one group [6]. Cases are allocated by residence in large administrative units

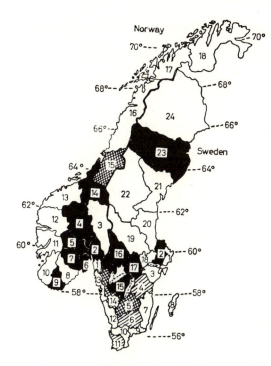

Fig. 4. Distribution of MS in Norway [8] and Sweden [9] by county of residence. Solid areas are significantly above ($X^2a > 4.0$) national mean prevalence rates, cross-hatched high but of dubious significance (X^2a 2.0–4.0), diagonal-lined insignificantly high ($X^2a < 2.0$), and open areas below the national mean rate. Reproduced with permission from Acta Neurologica Scandinavica [6].

(counties), and the distributions tested statistically for deviations from homogeneity [7]. All studies to be mentioned now were markedly non-random. MS in Norway was assessed from SWANK's survey of rural cases from 1935 to 1948 [8], and in Sweden from SÄLLSTRÖM's study of 1925–1934 [9]. Solid black areas are significantly above the national mean prevalence rate, cross-hatched ones high but of dubioussignificance, diagonal-lined regions insignificantly high, and open areas below the national mean (fig. 4). The same data can be classed in percentile ranges of the national prevalence rate (fig. 5). Note there is essentially a single cluster or focus of high frequency MS in Norway, and there seem to be two foci in Sweden.

Counties, especially in large countries, may not be the most desirable units to use to determine distributions because of their large or variable

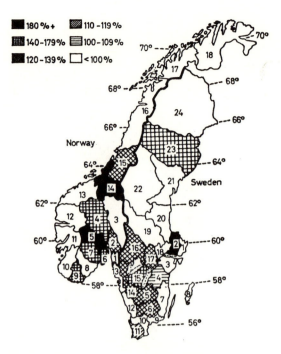

Fig. 5. Distribution of MS by county of residence in Norway [8] and Sweden [9], expressed as percentiles of the national mean prevalence rate in the ranges indicated on the map. Reproduced with permission from Archives of Neurology [2].

sizes and irregular outlines. Smaller administrative units are available for testing in Sweden (but not Norway), and are chosen in such a way that each unit would be expected to contain at least 5 cases of MS if the distribution were homogeneous [10]. In this fashion a more detailed picture of the distribution of MS can be defined (fig. 6). It can be seen we still have basically two foci, one on the northern coast near Umeå, and the major southern cluster. This one largely occupies the inland lake region and extends eastward to Uppsala (fig. 7).

The intensive study of MS in Denmark of 1950 by HYLLESTED [11] can be similarly delineated. Here the focus of MS by county extends across middle Jutland on to Funen (fig. 8). Again smaller administrative units can be used, and in this fashion basically the same findings are seen (fig. 9).

GEORGI and HALL [12] surveyed Switzerland in 1956, and the distribution of MS by county is also that of a single cluster, in the northwestern

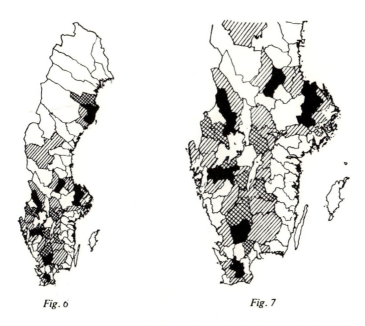

Fig. 6   *Fig. 7*

Fig. 6. Distribution of MS by small-unit residence in Sweden, as in figure 4. Reproduced with permission from Acta Neurologica Scandinavica [10].

Fig. 7. Distribution of MS by small units in southern Sweden, as in figure 6.

part of the country (fig. 10). Here too small units are available. Most of the high rate areas, and all those significantly high, fall within the same general region (Fig. 11). This may be looked upon as forming a rather irregular and somewhat discontinuous focus of high frequency MS (fig. 12).

We thus have evidence that MS is distributed in clusters or foci of cases in these high-frequency countries. In two instances there were earlier studies of the distribution of MS in the same countries. GRAM's survey [13] covered 1921–1934, and was almost identical with HYLLESTED's (fig. 13). ACKERMANN [14] and BING and REESE [15] evaluated the Swiss cases of 1918–1922, and again northwestern Switzerland was the site of the focus (fig. 14). In formal testing both countries showed a high coefficient of correlation, about 0.8, between the old and the new studies of MS (fig. 15). Recent prevalence studies in Norway by PRESTHUS [16] and by OFTEDAL [17, 18] also confirm SWANK's figures [8] for the regions surveyed. In view of this geographic stability, we can ignore the time differences between the studies and thus consider that the connection of high

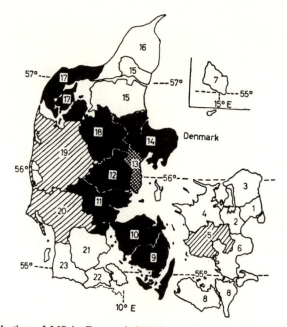

Fig. 8. Distribution of MS in Denmark [11] by county of residence, as in figure 4. Reproduced with permission from Acta Neurologica Scandinavica [6].

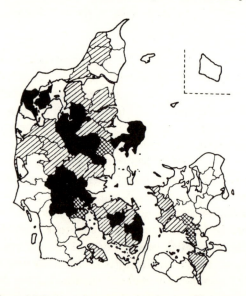

Fig. 9. Distribution of MS by small-unit residence in Denmark, as in figure 4. Reproduced with permission from Acta Neurologica Scandinavica [10].

94

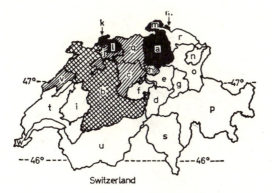

Fig. 10. Distribution of MS in Switzerland [12] by county of residence, as in figure 4. Reproduced with permission from Acta Neurologica Scandinavica [6].

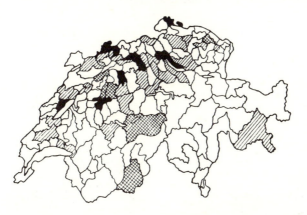

Fig. 11. Distribution of MS by small-unit residence in Switzerland, as in figure 4. Reproduced with permission from Acta Neurologica Scandinavica [10].

rate areas in the south between Norway and Sweden (fig. 4) can be interpreted as evidence of a single focus across both these countries. This leaves the northern Swedish focus still to be explained.

RINNE [19] has recently described the distribution of MS in Finland for 1964. The cases here too form a single cluster in the southwestern part of the country, as shown by County Hospital Districts (fig. 16). When we look at Fennoscandia together, it seems that Finland serves to link the two Swedish foci. Thus the clustering of MS by county appears to start in the southern plains of Norway, extend across the lake region of Sweden to

95

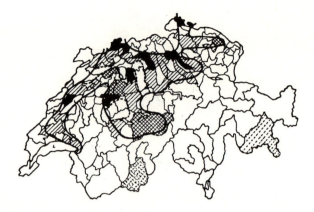

Fig. 12. Outline of 'focus' of MS in Switzerland from figure 11. Reproduced with permission from Acta Neurologica Scandinavica [10].

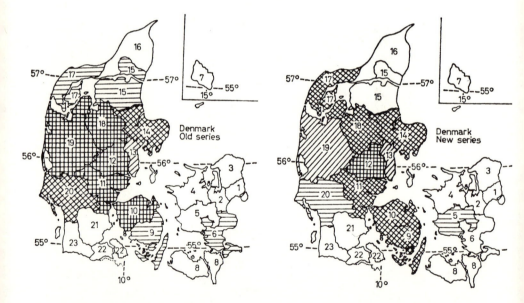

Fig. 13. Comparison of distributions of MS in Denmark by county from early [13] and later [11] studies for different generations of patients as percentiles of the mean. Reproduced with permission from Archives of Neurology [2].

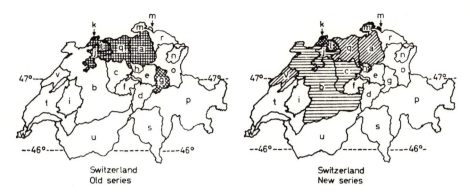

Fig. 14. Comparison of distributions of MS in Switzerland by county in early [14, 15] and later [12] studies for different generations of patients, as percentiles of the mean. Reproduced with permission from Archives of Neurology [2].

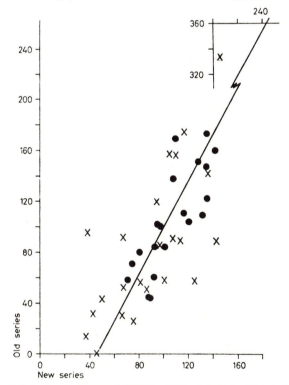

Fig. 15. Correlation of prevalence of MS by county between old and new studies of Denmark (●) and Switzerland (×) with each county noted as its percentages of the national mean prevalence rates. Reproduced with permission from Archives of Neurology [2].

97

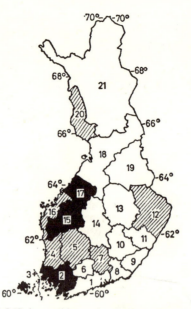

Fig. 16. Distribution of MS by residence in County Hospital District in Finland [19], as in figure 4. Reproduced with permission from Acta Neurologica Scandinavica [20].

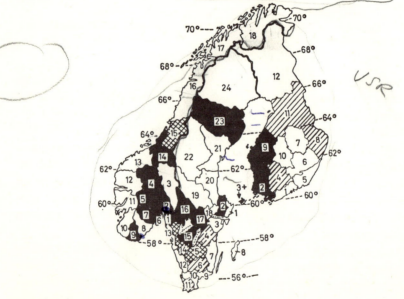

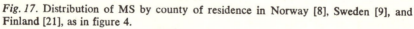

Fig. 17. Distribution of MS by county of residence in Norway [8], Sweden [9], and Finland [21], as in figure 4.

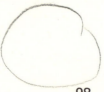

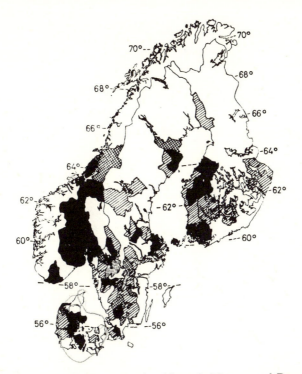

Fig. 18. Distribution of MS by county of residence in Norway and Denmark, County Hospital District in Finland, and small units in Sweden, as in figure 4.

Uppsala, and then to cross the Bay of Bothnia by way of Åland and go up the coast of Finland, returning to Sweden at Umeå (fig. 17). When the small units are utilized for the MS distributions, this impression of a single Fennoscandian focus of MS seems even more definite (fig. 18). This appears much too marked to blame on statistical artefact or coincidence. And none of these foci could be attributed to distributions of medical facilities [22]. On the basis of these findings, I believe that there must be an essential relationship of MS with some factor or factors of similar geographic distribution, and therefore that MS can be defined as an acquired exogenous disease.

If this be true, the next question is when is the disease acquired. Looking once more at HYLLESTED's study, we note that the cases of MS appear most concentrated in the period when the patients were less than 15 years of age (fig. 19). Even with age-specific rates for cases and population, this childhood period (A) looks more dense than the onset period (B)

99

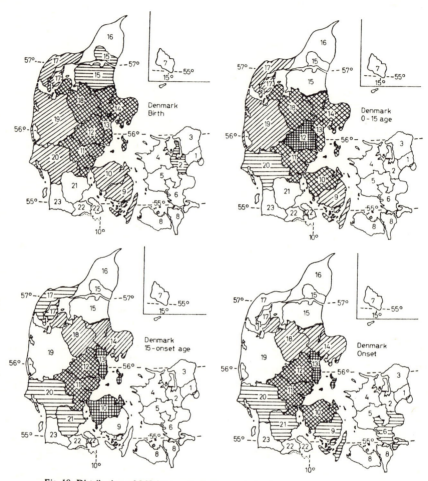

Fig. 19. Distribution of MS by county in Denmark for four life-periods in cases per total population, as percentiles of the national mean rate.

(fig. 20). For any exogenous illness, the greatest concentration of cases will occur at the time when the disease is acquired. From this viewpoint then, we might suspect that MS may well be acquired somewhere around

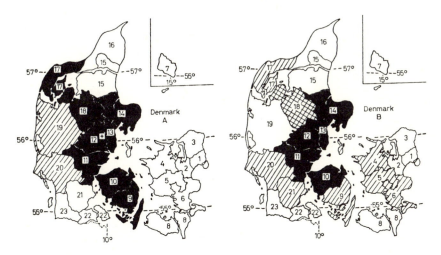

Fig. 20. Distribution of MS by county in Denmark during childhood (A) and at onset (B) as in figure 4, by age-specific prevalence rates. Reproduced with permission from Acta Neurologica Scandinavica [20].

the ages of 10 to 15 by natives of high frequency MS regions [23]. Fragmentary data in support of this are provided by the works of BAMMER [24], DEAN [25], ALTER [26], and WAINERDI [27]; and SCHAPIRA [28] independently arrived at the same inference by an ingenious study of sibs with MS.

With BEEBE, KURLAND, and others, an intensive evaluation of MS in US Army personnel in World War II has been under way for the past 11 years [4, 5]. Although all 762 men were classed as MS by the Army, we considered only ²/₃ to be MS, after reviewing all available follow-up data for the period to 1962 *(table I)*. Based on random service numbers, controls to these cases were then matched for age and length of service, and a large amount of data of epidemiologic interest assessed [4]. Of pertinence here are the times of residence *(table II)*. The marked north-south differential for residence at birth and induction had totally disappeared in the short months between induction and clinical onset. Indeed all differentiating features found for MS cases vs. controls pertained to events which antedated service, regardless of the time of clinical onset, and this study

101

Table I. Final diagnoses after review with 5 to 20 years follow-up for 762 men classed as multiple sclerosis in the Army in World War II, for the total series and the case-control epidemiologic series [4, 5]

Group	Dx	Total series No.	%	Epidemiologic series No.	%	group
1	(definite MS)[1]	476	62.4	353	61.6	} 'MS'
2A	(strong possible MS)	51	6.7	36	6.3	}
2B	(poor possible MS)	45	5.9	33	5.8	[2]
3	(not MS)	146	19.2	115	20.1	'not MS'
4	(unknown)	41	5.4	33	5.8	[2]
5	(primary lat. sclerosis)	3	0.4	3	0.5	[2]
	Total	762	100.0	573	100.1	

[1] Diagnostic criteria are essentially those of the SCHUMACHER committee [33].
[2] Discarded.

Table II. Residence by tier expressed as case-control ratios for MS cases at birth, at induction, and in service [1] in Army MS series [4]

Tier	Time of residence birth	induction	in service[1]
North	1.45	1.38	1.03
Middle	0.86	0.86	0.99
South	0.75	0.80	1.07
Total	1.01	1.00	1.03
N (cases)	373	388	578
P	<0.01	<0.01	>0.10

[1] Residences in service prior to clinical onset only.

therefore provides additional evidence of prolonged latency in this disease.

We had also evaluated a totally distinct series of Army men who had acute idiopathic optic neuropathy in World War II, and had found that only 12 % of these 183 men had progressed to MS in the ensuing 13–15 years [29]. Only high educational level and poor vision at induction seemed to be associated with such progression. However, when we look at

Table III. Residence at birth for MS cases from Army MS series [4], in case-control ratios

North-South tier	East-West blocks West	Central	East	Total	N
North	1.25	1.31	1.60	1.45	154
Middle	0.86	0.79	0.96	0.86	152
South	0.63	0.70	1.05	0.75	67
Total	0.85	0.88	1.22	1.01	
N	68	126	179		373

Table IV. Ratios for induction residence of cases observed/expected for optic neuropathy in separate Army series [29]

Region	Optic neuropathy
North East and North Central	1.14
South East and South Central	0.84
Montain-Pacific	0.68
Total	1.00
N	182
P	0.06

the entire optic neuropathy (O.N.) series, there are a number of interesting comparisons with the separate MS series already discussed. The birth place residences for the MS cases indicate in general a maximum risk in the northeastern US and lowest ratios in the southwest *(table III)*. The total O.N. group shows this same general relationship *(table IV)*. Birth and induction data are almost identical in these works, since they refer to the same locales in some 85 % of the men. One of the strongest differentiating features found in the MS was a positive association with high socioeconomic status, whether measured by occupational or educational levels. In *table V* are the educational levels expressed as percentage frequencies for each of these series, compared with those of the controls from the MS series. Note the equivalence of MS and O.N. rates. In similar fashion we see the ratios for visual acuity at induction for MS and O.N. cases *(table VI)*. In both, there is an excess of men with subnormal

Table V. Percentage frequency distribution for educational level of men with optic neuropathy and MS from separate Army series [4, 29]

Years	Optic Neuropathy [29]	MS [4]	Controls (MS+not-MS) [4]
<9	23.8	23.0	31.9
9–11	24.9	25.3	26.4
12	26.0	29.2	28.7
13≤	25.4	22.5	13.0
Total	100.1	100.0	100.0
N	181	387	499

Table VI. Ratios for induction visual acuity of cases observed/expected for optic neuropathy and cases-controls for MS from separate Army series of World War II [4, 29]

Visual acuity	Optic neuropathy [29]	MS [4]
–20/20	1.01	0.79
20/21–20/30	0.74	1.26
20/31+	1.28	1.55
Total	1.00	0.99
N	177	384
P	<0.01	<0.01

vision. We can also compare the age distributions of O.N. and MS *(table VII)*. Here again the O.N. and MS series are equivalent, and much different from the distribution of all enlisted men in service at that time. Lastly, the racial composition of the MS series was such that only 4 % of the MS cases were Negroes in contrast to an expected frequency of 11 %. Of the O.N. series, only 6 % were Negroes.

Thus, in all testable features the entire O.N. group was very similar to the separate MS series even though only 1 in 8 O.N. progressed to MS. This could be taken to indicate that both states are actually variants of one single disease. In the Army MS series [30] $1/_2$ of the Group A cases [4]

---

[4] Group A cases refer to those with an onset bout separate from the Army diagnostic bout, and I believe is close to representing the naturally-occurring clinical onset of MS in the general (male) population.

Table VII. Percentage frequency distribution for age at admission for cases of optic neuropathy and of MS in separate Army series [29, 30], versus 1943–1945 Army-wide distribution; all three for enlisted men only

Age	Optic neuropathy [29]	MS [30]	Enlisted men [29]
<20	2.8	3.6	9.0
20–24	33.6	27.3	40.0
25–29	28.0	29.8	27.5
30–34	26.0	24.5	14.7
35≤	9.3	14.8	8.9
Total	99.9	100.0	100.1
N	107	527	–

Table VIII. Frequency of type of symptom during the onset bout in Group A MS patients of Army MS series [30]

Type	Alone	Total[1]
	percentage	
Motor	12	40
Coordination	5	27
Sensory	9	34
Brain Stem	19	34
Visual	7	28
Average	10	–
Σ 4 other types	<1	–
Total	52	97
N	293	

[1] this type alone or with others

of MS had an onset bout characterized by a single type of symptom (motor, coordination, sensory, brain stem, visual) (table VIII). If each of the other single-type onsets showed the same progression rate as O.N., one would need 5,000 cases to provide 625 'classical' MS. The multiple-type onsets would add 625 more for a total of 5,625 cases of 'true' MS, out of which only 1,250 would be recognized as 'classical' MS. This is a ratio of 4.5 to 1. If we take simply the O.N. progression rate and assume this represents all MS onsets, the ratio of 'true' to 'classical' MS would be 8 to 1.

Table IX. Correlations of MS distributions with those of childhood diseases [31]

Disease	Year	During childhood years			During prevalence years		
		Norway	Denmark	Switzerland	Norway	Denmark	Switzerland
Measles	1	(—++)	(—+)	+	(—+)	0	0
	2	0	0	0	0	0	+
	3	+	0	0	+	0	0
	4	0	+	++	—	—	+
	total	+	0	0	0	0	++
Mumps	1	0	+	0	(—++)	0	0
	2	0	0	+	0	0	+
	3	0	0	0	0	0	0
	4	0	(—+)	0	—	—	++
	total	0	0	0	0	0	+
Scarlatina	1	0	+	+	0	0	++
	2	0	0	+	—	—	++
	3	0	+	+	—	—	++
	4	0	0	+	—	0	++
	total	0	+	+	0	0	++
Diphtheria	1	0	0	+	—	—	—
	2	0	0	0			
	3	0	0	+			
	4	0	0	+			
	total	0	0	+	—	—	—
Pertussis	1	0	0	0	—	—	—
	2	++	0	0			
	3	0	0	++			
	4	+	0	+			
	total	++	0	0	—	—	—

+ significant correlation 5 % level.
++ significant correlation 1 % level.
(—++) *negative* correlation significant at 1 % level.
0 no correlation at 5 % level.
— not tested.

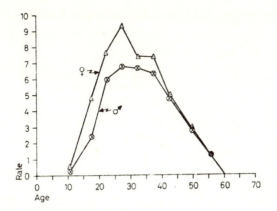

Fig. 21. Average annual age-specific incidence rates for MS in Denmark [11], in cases per 100,000 population.

Thus the 'true' prevalence of MS could well be 4 to 8 times as great as we believe, or as high as 4 MS per 1000 population in the high frequency MS band. This has special relevance to the consideration of an infectious origin for MS, against which concept has been the rarity of the disease, with too small a reservoir of afflicted persons to maintain the disease in a population. And if transmissibility persisted during life after either clinical or hypothetical onset, the man-years of exposure would further be greatly magnified, even though acquisition of disease were limited to the young.

There are two other epidemiologic features of MS which could be compatible with an infectious origin. In an intensive comparison of the distributions of many diseases with those of MS [31], the only notable positive associations found were for childhood infectious diseases *(table IX)*. Measles showed intermittently a moderate correlation for the years when the MS prevalence studies were done, as well as for the years when the MS patients were children. In similar fashion, mumps, and more strongly scarlatina, demonstrated this relationship. Pertussis and diphtheria in childhood also at times showed moderate correlations. Dr. SEVER's data [32] on serum antibodies in MS also might suggest an infectious origin. The last point to consider is the shape of the curve which represents the age-specific annual incidence rates for MS calculated from the data of HYLLESTED (fig. 21). Note the steep rise, the short plateau, and the less rapid decline. A curve like this is reminiscent of acute infectious disease with long-lasting immunity. To be typical of many acute infections, the curve should be moved to the left some 10 or 15 years, which again might be considered to support the concept of latency, as well as the possibility of an infectious origin.

While these data would be *compatible* with infection, it is obvious there are many other types of exogenous agents which have to be considered, even if one grants that MS may well be an exogenous disease. Exogenous factors of 'animal, vegetable, or mineral' origin must be entertained – and this has not yet been attempted in this context. It is not too improbable that further investigation might lead along an entirely different trail from infection, and at our present state of ignorance, no clue can be ignored. An infectious origin also is by no means a leading or even a serious contender in the minds of many workers. Epidemiologic inferences are at best circumstantial, and rest upon quite tangential evidence. The only acceptable proof of an infectious cause for MS can be the isolation or transmission of such an agent on a regular basis from cases of MS, which of course has not been accomplished. Therefore an infectious origin for MS must remain, at present, no more than an interesting hypothesis deserving the Scottish verdict of 'not proven'.

References

1. KURTZKE, J. F.: General features of the prevalence of multiple sclerosis. J. Indian med. Prof. *11:* 4896–4901, 4895 (1964).
2. KURTZKE, J. F.: An epidemiologic approach to multiple sclerosis. Arch. Neurol. *14:* 213–222 (1966).
3. STAZIO, A. and KURLAND, L. T.: Multiple sclerosis: its frequency and distribution with special reference to Washington, D. C. Neurology *12:* 445–452 (1962).
4. BEEBE, G. W.; KURTZKE, J. F.; KURLAND, L. T.; AUTH, T. L. and NAGLER, B.: Studies on the natural history of multiple sclerosis. 3. Epidemiologic analysis of the Army experience in World War II. Neurology *17:* 1–17 (1967).
5. NAGLER, B.; BEEBE, G. W.; KURTZKE, J. F.; KURLAND, L. T.; AUTH, T. L. and NEFZGER, M. D.: Studies on the natural history of multiple sclerosis. 1. Design and diagnosis. Acta neurol. scand. *42:* suppl. 19, 141–156 (1966).
6. KURTZKE, J. F.: An evaluation of the geographic distribution of multiple sclerosis. Acta neurol. scand. *42:* suppl. 19, 91–117 (1966).
7. KURTZKE, J. F.: On statistical testing of prevalence studies. J. chron. Dis. *19:* 909–922 (1966).
8. SWANK, R. L.; LERSTAD, O.; STRØM, A. and BACKER, J.: Multiple sclerosis in rural Norway. Its geographic and occupational incidence in relation to nutrition. New Engl. J. Med. *246:* 721–728 (1952).
9. SÄLLSTRÖM, T.: Das Vorkommen und die Verbreitung der multiplen Sklerose in Schweden. Zur geographischen Pathologie der multiplen Sklerose. Acta med. scand., suppl. *137:* 1–141 (1942).
10. KURTZKE, J. F.: On the fine structure of the distribution of multiple sclerosis. Acta neurol. scand. *43:* 257–282 (1967).

11. HYLLESTED, K.: Disseminated sclerosis in Denmark. Prevalence and geographical distribution. (Rosenkilde & Bagger, Copenhagen 1956).
12. GEORGI, F.; HALL, P. und MÜLLER, H. R.: Zur Problematik der multiplen Sklerose. Geomedizinische Studien in der Schweiz und in Ost-Afrika und ihre Bedeutung für Ätiologie und Pathogenese. Bibl. psychiat. neurol. *114:* 1–123 (1961).
13. GRAM, H. C.: Den disseminerede skleroses forekomst i Danmark. Ugeskr. Laeg. *96:* 823–825 (1934).
14. ACKERMANN, A.: Die multiple Sklerose in der Schweiz. Enquête von 1918–22. Schweiz. med. Wschr. *61:* 1245–1250 (1931).
15. BING, R. und REESE, H.: Die multiple Sklerose in der Nordwestschweiz (Kantone Basel, Solothurn, Aargau, Luzern). Schweiz. med. Wschr. *56:* 30–34 (1926).
16. PRESTHUS, J.: Multiple sclerosis in Møre og Romsdal County, Norway. Acta neurol. scand. *42:* suppl. 19, 12–18 (1966).
17. OFTEDAL, S.: Discussion at geomedical conference. Acta psychiat. neurol. scand. *35:* suppl. 147, 98–99 (1960).
18. OFTEDAL, S.-I.: Multiple sclerosis in Vestfold, Norway. Acta neurol. scand. *42:* suppl. 19, 19–26 (1966) (also ibid *41:* suppl. 16, 1965).
19. RINNE, U. K.; PANELIUS, M.; KIVALO, E.; HOKKANEN, E. and PALO, J.: Distribution of multiple sclerosis in Finland, with special reference to some geological factors. Acta neurol. scand. *42:* 385–399 (1966).
20. KURTZKE, J. F.: Further considerations on the geographic distribution of multiple sclerosis. Acta neurol. scand. *43:* 283–298 (1967).
21. RINNE, U. K.: Personal communication, April 17, 1967.
22. KURTZKE, J. F.: Medical facilities and the prevalence of multiple sclerosis. Acta neurol. scand. *41:* 561–579 (1965).
23. KURTZKE, J. F.: On the time of onset in multiple sclerosis. Acta neurol. scand. *41:* 140–158 (1965).
24. BAMMER, H.: Felduntersuchungen über die Verbreitung der Multiplen Sklerose im Spessart und dem benachbarten Siedlungsraum. Münch. med. Wschr. *102:* 1115–1119 (1960).
25. DEAN, G.: Disseminated sclerosis in South Africa. Its relationship to swayback disease and suggested treatment. Brit. med. J. *1:* 842–845 (1949).
26. ALTER, M.; LEIBOWITZ, U. and SPEER, J.: Risk of multiple sclerosis related to age at immigration to Israel. Arch. neurol. *15:* 234–237 (1966).
27. WAINERDI, H. R.: Does the multiple-sclerosis syndrome begin at puberty? Boston med. Quart. *12:* 44–47 (1961).
28. SCHAPIRA, K.; POSKANZER, D. C. and MILLER, H.: Familial and conjugal multiple sclerosis. Brain *86:* 315–332 (1963).
29. KURLAND, L. T.; BEEBE, G. W.; KURTZKE, J. F.; NAGLER, B.; AUTH, T. L.; LESSELL, S. and NEFZGER, M. D.: Studies on the natural history of multiple sclerosis. 2. The progression of optic neuritis to multiple sclerosis. Acta neurol. scand. *42:* suppl. 19, 157–176 (1966).
30. KURTZKE, J. F.; BEEBE, G. W.; NAGLER, B.; AUTH, T. L.; KURLAND, L. T. and NEFZGER, M. D.: Studies on the natural history of multiple sclerosis. 4. Clinical features of the onset bout. Acta neurol. scand. in press.
31. KURTZKE, J. F.: The distribution of multiple sclerosis and other diseases. Acta neurol. scand. *42:* 221–243 (1966).
32. REED, D.; SEVER, J.; KURTZKE, J. and KURLAND, L.: Measles antibody in patients with multiple sclerosis. Arch. Neurol. *10:* 402–410 (1964).
33. SCHUMACHER, G. A. *et al.*: Problems of experimental trials of therapy in multiple sclerosis: report by the panel on the evaluation of experimental trials of therapy in multiple sclerosis. Ann. N. Y. Acad. Sci. *122:* 552–568 (1965).

Involvement of the Immune Mechanism

Cerebrospinal Fluid Proteins and Serum Immunoglobulins

Occurrence in Multiple Sclerosis and Other Neurological Diseases: Comparative Measurement of γ-Globulin and the IgG Class

Mariella Fischer-Williams, MD, and Ronald C. Roberts, PhD

T EN YEARS ago, Smith et al suggested that multiple sclerosis (MS) may be an autoimmune disease characterized by delayed hypersensitivity, but data have not yet provided the proof. To improve the diagnosis of MS and throw some light on its pathogenesis, we studied the proteins in the cerebrospinal fluid (CSF) and the serum. By so doing, we sought to differentiate between neurologic diseases in which (1) the blood-CSF barrier is intact, (2) the blood-CSF barrier is temporarily impaired, and (3) immunoglobulins in the central nervous system are altered.

The electroimmunodiffusion (EID) method of Hartley et al reliably measures specific proteins in small samples of unconcentrated CSF. Using this method for the immunoglobulin class G (IgG), Schneck and

Claman obtained results comparable to those reported by Kabat et al for the classical immune precipitation technique.

We compared the IgG concentrations measured by EID with γ-globulin concentrations measured by cellulose-acetate electrophoresis of CSF concentrates, the latter a common method in clinical laboratories.

The quantitative changes in proteins (particularly the immunoglobulins) of the blood and the CSF in MS were compared with changes in other patients with neurological disease and in a group of anxiety patients considered as "controls."

Previous detailed studies[3-11] have shown that the practical diagnostic significance of CSF protein analysis appears to revolve around only two determinations, the total proteins and the immunoglobulin levels. Of

112

the immunoglobulins, only IgG seems diagnostically important. Levels of γ-globulin or IgG reported as a percentage of the total CSF proteins are useful in the diagnosis of MS, postexanthematous and postvaccinial "allergic" (or "autoimmune") encephalomyelitis, neurosyphilis, and subacute sclerosing panencephalitis (SSPE).[12]

Materials and Methods

The CSF and sera from 334 patients with a variety of neurological disorders (Fig 1) were obtained by lumbar puncture and blood drawn on the same day.

The total protein was estimated by the trichloroacetic acid turbidometric method of Meulemans.[13] Using this technique, the upper limit of normal was 55 mg/100 ml and the coefficient of variation 4.8%.

The CSF was concentrated to one drop (0.05 to 0.1 ml) in preparation for cellulose acetate electrophoresis by ultrafiltration against reduced pressure through collodion membranes as described by Whitaker and Lemmi.[14] The procedure was done at room temperature, and the initial volume of CSF to be concentrated was determined by dividing 1.82 by the initial protein concentration in milligrams per milliliter. The recovery efficiency of electrophoretic fractions after concentration was tested by diluting normal serum of known electrophoretic composition 200 times with physiological saline and then concentrating it by the same procedure. Duplicate determinations indicated losses of 1.3% in the gamma fraction and none in the other fractions.

Electrophoresis of the CSF concentrates was performed on 1 × 6-inch cellulose acetate strips in tromethamine (Tris)-barbital buffer, 0.05 ionic strength at pH 8.8 and 300 for 45 minutes. The various fractions were quantitated by densitometry.

Cerebrospinal fluid IgG was assayed in 5-microliter samples of unconcentrated CSF by EID. Minimum levels of detection of IgG were approximately 1.0 mg/100 ml CSF for all runs. For statistical analyses we assumed all undetectable IgG levels to be 1.0 mg/100 ml. Because discussion centers on high levels of IgG, this does not influence our conclusions.

We used commercially available kits to assay serum IgG, IgA, and IgM by the radial immunodiffusion method of Mancini et al.[15]

Results

The results on the CSF and sera were analyzed for 21 diagnostic categories. Significant differences between the groups were found in the electrophoretic gamma fraction and in the IgG of the CSF and are therefore discussed. Since no significant differences were observed in any of the other CSF protein fractions (prealbumin, albumin, α_1, α_2, and β-globulins), nor in the IgG and IgM in the serum, the findings are not reported. The serum IgA is discussed in order to compare our results with published data.

Cerebrospinal Fluid.—The *gamma electrophoretic fraction* was expressed as percent of total protein (Fig 1). In all the figures, the total length of the bar represents the range of values, with the mean at the interface between the *solid* and the *hatched*. This illustrates the skewness of distribution in many of the categories. The mean is shifted towards the end of the bar with the higher density of data, and a *long hatched* part shows that few cases fell above the mean. The highest mean and most of the high levels were found in MS patients, and the differences between them and all other neurological cases were highly significant ($P > 0.001$). In the "possible" MS group, the mean gamma fraction was higher (but not significantly so) than in all other categories except viral meningoencephalitis. The patients with anxiety but no other detectable neurological disease were taken as "controls," and the highest level of their gamma fraction was 13.4%. From these findings and those of Hartley et al[2] with IgG we adopted 14% of the total protein as the upper limit of normal. With this criterion, 94% (32 of 34) of the MS patients had a γ-globulin fraction which exceeded 14%, while only 7.7% (22 of 284) of all the non-MS patients had gamma fractions over 14%. Of these 22 patients, three had subarachnoid hemorrhage, two viral meningoencephalitis, two focal seizures, five miscellaneous neurological disease (optic nerve arachnoiditis, hepatic encephalopathy, cerebral edema, aseptic meningitis, and cerebral atrophy), and ten each had some other disease. In the "possible" MS group, 54% (7 of 13) had gamma fractions greater than 14%.

The IgG was determined by the EID method, and the results are shown in Fig 2 in the same way as in Fig 1. Comparison shows the much wider spread of IgG values

(Fig 2) obtained for all categories than of the gamma fraction (Fig 1). Multiple sclerosis patients had the highest mean IgG values of all the groups, followed by viral meningoencephalitis, subarachnoid hemorrhage, and the "possible" MS group. These groups had mean IgG levels exceeding 14% of the total protein.

The IgG values for the anxiety patients showed a skewed distribution with 15 of them below 13% but with individual values of 28% and 26% with total protein of 14 mg and 20 mg, respectively. We adopted 14% of the upper limit of normal because of the prior observations of Hartley et al[2] in a group of "normals" larger than ours. The occasional high IgG value associated with low total protein in patients with anxiety and with no other detected disease is puzzling. Perhaps the IgG method is unreliable when the total protein level is below 20 mg/100 ml, or perhaps biochemical deviations were present in these anxiety patients. Considering 14% IgG as the upper limit of normal, 75% of the MS patients had IgG levels exceeding 14%, while 23% of the non-MS group had IgG levels greater than 14%. The majority of these "false positive" patients had viral meningoencephalitis, (3/7), focal seizures (10/32), miscellaneous neurological disease (12/35), or cerebral arteriosclerosis (5/23). One third of the false positive patients had total CSF proteins less than 20 mg/100 ml.

CSF Total Proteins.—The mean CSF total protein was highest in the MS group, except for the Guillain-Barré syndrome. The mean for MS was 48 mg/100 ml, with seven cases between 55 and 82 mg/100 ml and one exceptionally low at 10 mg/100 ml. In the controls the mean and standard deviation was 28 ± 8.2 mg/100 ml, which is close to the normal range reported for this assay. In the Guillain-Barré patients the mean and standard deviation were 270 ± 167 mg/100 ml.

CSF Electrophoretic Fractions Other Than Gamma.—Analysis of the electrophoretic fractions other than the gamma fraction in the various disease categories showed no distinct or diagnostic features. The only paraprotein band was observed in a patient with IgG multiple myeloma.

Serum.—The results on IgA are reported because Uyeda et al[16] detected significantly higher levels in patients with MS than with other neurological disorders. The mean and standard deviation of the serum IgA levels in the MS group were 218 ± 114 mg/100 ml, while in all the other patients in this series the corresponding values were 231 ± 140 mg/100 ml. The difference between the means is not significant.

Serum IgG/CSF IgG Ratio (or "Index"). —The ratio of serum IgG to CSF IgG was examined in the various groups (Fig 3). The index plotted on the x-axis was obtained by dividing the CSF IgG into the serum IgG for each patient, giving the number of times more IgG in serum than in CSF. Figure 3 shows that this index was highest in the controls (the anxiety group) and lowest in the MS group except for Guillain-Barré polyneuropathy cases. Here the serum IgG/CSF IgG ratio was extremely low, because all CSF proteins over 70 mg/100 ml were infrequent and did not influence the serum IgG/CSF IgG index.

Comment

With certain differences, our findings confirm many of the positive and negative results of other recent authors whose questions were presumably similar to ours.

The establishment of criteria for the clinical diagnosis of MS is a constant source of discussion.[17] The patients in this series were under the personal care of one of us (MF-W) or of one of the other members of the Neurology Department of the Marshfield Clinic. The clinical diagnosis was made when there was dissemination in time and anatomical distribution plus a history of relapses and remissions. Cases in which the history was steadily progressive and those without evidence of multiple sites for the pathogenesis of physical signs were either rejected or placed in the group of "possible MS." Patients with retrobulbar neuritis alone were also classified as "possible MS."

It is of technical importance to determine which method of measurement gives the highest percentage of positive results in MS and the lowest of false positives in cases other than MS.

Using paper electrophoresis and concentrated CSF, Schapira and Park[6] found ele-

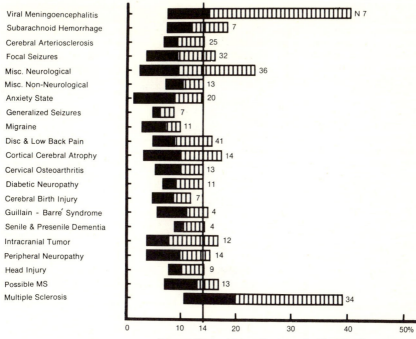

Fig 1.—Gamma electrophoretic fractions in CSF expressed as percent of total protein found in various disease categories. Total length of **bar** represents range of values found. Interface between the **solid** and **hatched** is mean. **Number** on the right indicates number of patients in each category.

vated γ-globulin in 88% of 81 MS patients, and Cosgrove and Agius[8] found it raised in 80% of 153 patients with MS, (15.9 ± 7.5%).

With the immunochemical (quantitative precipitin) method of Kabat and others,[4] Yahr et al[5] found raised γ-globulin in 66.5% of 244 cases of MS and in 74% of 35 cases of neurosyphilis, and Tourtellotte[7] found raised γ-globulins (12.9% ± 2.1%) in 50% of 387 MS cases.

With the radial diffusion technique, Riddoch and Thompson[9] found IgG raised to a mean of 19% of total CSF proteins in 62% of 45 cases of MS, compared with 14% of 160 patients with various other neurological disorders.

Using agar gel electrophoresis in a qualitative study, Laterre et al[10] in the largest series so far reported (2,043 patients) found a "peculiar" γ-globulin pattern in 75.2% to

86.9% of 323 MS patients. A similar abnormal or peculiar pattern was observed in 39.6% of 144 other patients with inflammatory disease of the central nervous system (CNS) (encephalitis or meningoencephalitis of presumed or proven viral origin, bacterial meningitis or aseptic meningitis and abscess, neurosyphilis, toxoplasmosis, and in all eight cases of SSPE). In a previous quantitative study in 1966 using agar gel electrophoresis, Laterre had found γ-globulin raised in 72% of MS patients, but his top normal was only 10%.

Using the EID method, Schneck and Claman[3] found 56% of 54 MS patients with a level of IgG above 14%. Also using EID, Takase and Yoshida[18] found raised IgG in three cases of MS (with a mean of 10.6%), in three cases of tuberculous meningitis (14.4%), and in four cases of neurosyphilis (21.2%).

115

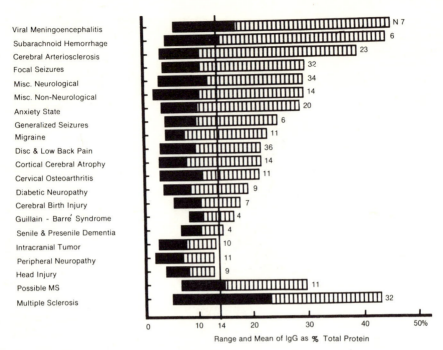

Viral Meningoencephalitis N 7
Subarachnoid Hemorrhage 6
Cerebral Arteriosclerosis 23
Focal Seizures 32
Misc. Neurological 34
Misc. Non-Neurological 14
Anxiety State 20
Generalized Seizures 6
Migraine 11
Disc & Low Back Pain 36
Cortical Cerebral Atrophy 14
Cervical Osteoarthritis 11
Diabetic Neuropathy 9
Cerebral Birth Injury 7
Guillain - Barré Syndrome 4
Senile & Presenile Dementia 4
Intracranial Tumor 10
Peripheral Neuropathy 11
Head Injury 9
Possible MS 11
Multiple Sclerosis 32

0   10 14   20   30   40   50%

Range and Mean of IgG as % Total Protein

Fig 2.—Range and mean of IgG concentrations in CSF expressed as percent of total protein for disease categories. See Fig 1 for further details.

It would seem of theoretical importance in the pathogenesis of MS to determine which index is the most sensitive for this disease. In the serum most of the γ-globulins are immunoglobulins. Thus, the globulins associated with immune processes tend to overlap or fall into the class of γ-globulins with a certain electrical charge, but the two categories are not superimposable. This distinction holds true for the CSF globulins, because Laterre et al[19] showed that most of the CSF immunoglobulins have the same antigenic determinants as serum immunoglobulins.

Few authors have used more than one method on the same CSF sample except to compare colloidal curves with one of the newer techniques. Schneck and Claman[3] believe that "if the measurement of CSF immunoglobulins is to be meaningful, these fractions [or subfractions of the γ-globulin] should be quantitated separately." In our series, however, estimation of the entire gamma fraction was a more sensitive index for

MS in that it showed closer correlation with clinical MS than estimation of the subfraction IgG. Thus, in 94% of our cases, the gamma fraction was more than 14% of the CSF total protein, whereas with the EID method the IgG was more than 14% in only 75% of our cases and only 56% of Schneck and Claman's patients. The gamma fraction also gave fewer false positives in MS. In 284 patients who did not have clinical MS, there were 7.7% with a gamma fraction above 14% of the total CSF proteins, where 23% of these patients showed IgG levels above 14%. (Fig 1 and 2). It may be, however, that these fractions and subfractions are associated with different processes or different stages of the disease.

Using agar gel electrophoresis and immunoelectrophoresis, van Welsum and van der Helm[20] found increased γ-globulin (up to 45%) and increased IgG and IgA in two out of five patients with subacute necrotizing encephalitis. Both patients had a protracted

116

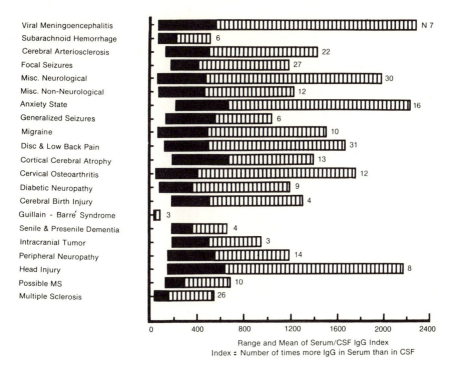

Fig 3.—Serum IgG/CSF IgG ratios (or "index") by disease category. Range and mean of "index" are presented as in Fig 1 and 2 for each category. Note that order of disease categories is different from that in Fig 1 and 2.

course (one died 16 months after onset of illness and the other recovered clinically in four months), as opposed to normal or negative results in three acute cases, verified by autopsy, which were fatal in two or three weeks.

The duration of the disease may therefore play a part, with normal or negative results in the acute phase, and abnormal or positive results in the subacute phase. We have not seen reported, nor have we ourselves done serial CSF sampling in the same patients. This could be informative, but may not be justifiable. The evidence in the literature for correlation of results with disease stage in MS is conflicting and the question unresolved.

No significant feature in respect to age, sex, pregnancy, duration of disease, acuteness, or chronicity at the time of the CSF examination was noted in our series. Most of

the 34 MS cases were in the early stages, many of them receiving initial diagnosis. However, transient episodes, particularly retrobulbar neuritis, had frequently occurred several years before CSF examination.

Yahr et al[5] believed there was a correlation between the elevated gamma fraction in CSF and repeated attacks of MS, as well as with multiple lesions and marked functional disability. However, they could not correlate the gamma fraction with the type of onset, course, duration, or occurrence of new symptoms.

The MS cases in our study were divided into those with CSF total protein value above and below 50 mg/100 ml. There was no difference in the gamma fraction or the IgG percentages of the total CSF protein between the two groups. Kabat et al[4] found that more of their patients had a higher percentage of the gamma fraction when the total protein level was above 50 mg/100 ml. However, Schneck and Claman[3] found the opposite, which they attributed to earlier diagnosis and less severe disease.

We agree with Schneck and Claman[3] that the EID method may be less reliable if the total CSF protein is less than 20 mg/100 ml. This difficulty may arise in children with low CSF total protein and account for some of our false positives in the focal seizure patients and the anxiety group.

The EID method has the technical advantage of requiring only ten microliters of un-concentrated CSF provided it is not contaminated. The method is therefore useful when CSF is insufficient for the cellulose acetate procedure. In CNS diseases, the serum/CSF ratio may indicate whether in the blood-CSF barrier is intact or temporarily impaired, or whether excess or different immunoglobulin was formed within the CSF. The serum/CSF IgG ratio was significantly altered only in MS and "possible" MS patients, in the Guillain-Barré syndrome, and in subarachnoid hemorrhage. The very high CSF protein in Guillain-Barré polyneuropathy without a rise in serum IgG inevitably causes a marked drop in the ratio. The blood-CSF barrier may also be abnormal in some cases of this heterogenous syndrome. Three patients with subarachnoid hemorrhage had false positive CSF IgG levels. One of these had multiple myeloma with a high IgG in the serum and an impaired blood-CSF barrier in that the myeloma "M" spike appeared in the CSF.

Viral meningoencephalitis was the only other condition in which both the gamma fraction and the IgG percentages were above 14% of the total CSF protein. Similar high percentages have been noted by other authors in SSPE[12] and in neurosyphilis[5]; and a high gamma fraction in a few patients with phenothiazine or alcohol intoxication or a "schizophrenic picture with extrapyramidal disturbance."[21] In our series, MS can be differentiated from viral meningoencephalitis by the serum to CSF/IgG ratio, which in MS is pathologically low.

High γ-globulin was also noted in the CSF in certain cases with γ-globulin raised in the serum (such as periarteritis nodosa and Behçet's disease[5]) and in isolated neurological cases with normal serum γ-globulin.[5]

Apart from the positive features already discussed, there was no significant correlation in our series between disease entities and CSF electrophoretic patterns. Review of the literature suggests that this has largely been the experience of other workers. Electrophoretic morphology of γ-globulin in CSF was correlated with grading of physical disability in 2,043 neurological patients by Laterre et al.[10] Special electrophoretic patterns are described in their 323 patients with MS and in inflammatory CNS disease (viral encephalitis, bacterial meningitis, neurosyphilis, and SSPE), but in only 2% to 5% of the rest of the entire series was correlation noted.

On examination of immunoglobulins IgG, IgA, and IgM, the present findings in serum differ from those of certain authors. Pathological increased IgA levels were not found in the sera of MS patients, as reported by Uyeda et al.[16] Kolar et al[11] found "elevation or abnormal decrease in the serum IgA or IgM" or both in 26.2% of their 64 MS patients in a detailed survey of 37 aspects of the pathophysiology of serum and CSF immunoglobulins. They concluded (and we agree) that "no specific manifestations were observed which might allow per se the diagnosis of multiple sclerosis."

It would appear therefore that large surveys of CSF and serum proteins using the commonly available techniques of protein analysis probably will not yield more information of diagnostic significance.

We believe, however, that various avenues of research promise to bear fruit. The first relates to the formation of abnormal IgG within the CNS, Tourtellotte and Parker[22] found a positive correlation between the concentration of IgG in plaques of demyelination due to MS (as well as in white matter of normal appearance) and the concentration of this globulin in the CSF. In 11 cases of MS, the CSF was examined in life and at autopsy, and the brain was studied at autopsy; the increase of IgG in CSF appeared to reflect excess IgG in the brain.

Increased IgG concentration was also demonstrated in brain extracts in SSPE,[23] in Huntington's chorea, and in multiple myeloma.[24] Further studies on the localization of IgG within the CNS, together with studies of the blood-brain barrier and of the abnormal immunological processes in these diseases should throw light on pathogenesis. Using radioactive sodium and bromide, Bourdillon et al[25] did not demonstrate consistent abnormality in the blood-brain barrier in MS, but Haerer et al,[26] using sodium bromide, believed there was a significant lowering in MS with chronic disease deteriorating over two years or lasting more than ten years.

In 1961, Smith et al[1] concluded from a study with intrathecal tuberculin that MS was likely to be an autoimmune disease. Autosensitive may be a better term, and the delayed hypersensitivity may affect many parts of the body as well as the CNS. Further studies have now suggested the possible myelinolytic role of lymphocytes and of atypical mononuclear cells. Lymphocytes isolated from the sera of 31 MS patients showed increased transformation responses to human brain protein; compared with 28 control subjects,[27] this suggested specific lymphocyte sensitization. However, both positive[28] and negative[29] results have been reported with lymphocyte transformation.

Carnegie's recent demonstration[30] of the encephalitogenic protein of human brain represents a major advance and a chemical breakthrough. He has described the amino acid sequence of this basic protein and identified the encephalitogenic locus of this protein, which is contained in a peptide having the sole tryptophan residue. This highly encephalitogenic peptide may therefore soon be available for the production of experimental autoimmune encephalomyelitis, the "model" for demyelinating disease. We may therefore be rather nearer solving the riddle of this enigmatic disease identified by Charcot in 1868.

Conclusions

We determined the CSF γ-globulin (as a percentage of the total proteins) by cellulose acetate electrophoresis and compared the results with quantitative levels of IgG obtained by the EID method in 334 patients with a variety of neurological disease. These results were compared with those obtained in 20 patients with anxiety but no detectable neurological disease. Serum IgG, IgA, and IgM concentrations were determined for all patients from samples drawn on the same day as the CSF.

The values of the whole gamma fractions showed better correlation with clinical MS than IgG values obtained by the EID method. In 94% of our 34 patients with clinical MS, the gamma fraction was above 14% of the total CSF proteins. In 75% of these cases, the IgG class was more than 14%.

The EID method has the technical advantage of requiring only ten *micro*liters of unconcentrated CSF.

Meningoencephalitis of viral or presumed viral origin was the only other disease in our series in which significantly raised γ-globulin or IgG was found. We did not confirm previous reports of significant differences in serum IgA levels between patients with MS and those with other neurological disease or with anxiety.

The decreased ratio of serum IgG to CSF IgG in MS, as compared with the other patients in this series, supports the views of Tourtellotte[22] and other authors that excess IgG arises within the CNS.

The members of the Department of Neurological Sciences of the Marshfield Clinic referred the patients; Karen Hanson and John Folz gave technical assistance; Carolyn Sonnentag helped with data compilation.

References

1. Smith HV, Hughes IE, Hunter G: Intrathecal tuberculin in disseminated sclerosis: The immunological aspects. *J Neurol Neurosurg Psychiat* **24**:101-117, 1961.
2. Hartley TF, Merrill DA, Claman HN: Quantitation of immunoglobulins in cerebrospinal fluid. *Arch Neurol* **15**:472-479, 1966.
3. Schneck SA, Claman HN: CSF immunoglobulins in multiple sclerosis and other neurologic diseases: Measurement of electroimmunodiffusion. *Arch Neurol* **20**:132-139, 1969.
4. Kabat EA, Glusman M, Knaub U: Quantitative estimation of the albumin and gamma globulin in normal and pathologic cerebrospinal fluid by immunochemical methods. *Amer J Med* **4**:653-662, 1948.
5. Yahr MD, Goldensohn SS, Kabat EA: Further studies on the gamma globulin content of cerebrospinal fluid in multiple sclerosis and other neurological diseases. *Ann NY Acad Sci* **58**:613-624, 1954.
6. Schapira K, Park DE: Gamma globulin studies in multiple sclerosis and their application to the problem of diagnosis. *J Neurol Neurosurg Psychiat* **24**:121-124, 1961.
7. Tourtellotte WW: Multiple sclerosis and cerebrospinal fluid. *Med Clin N Amer* **47**:1619-1628, 1963.
8. Cosgrove JBR, Agius P: Studies in multiple sclerosis: II. Comparison of the beta-gamma globulin ratio, gamma globulin elevation, and first-zone colloidal gold curve in the cerebrospinal fluid. *Neu-*

rology **16**:197-204, 1966.

9. Riddoch D, Thompson RA: Immunoglobulin levels in the cerebrospinal fluid. *Brit Med J* **1**:396-399, 1970.

10. Laterre EC, Callewaert A, Heremans JF, et al: Electrophoretic morphology of gamma globulins in cerebrospinal fluid of multiple sclerosis and other diseases of the nervous system. *Neurology* **20**:982-990, 1970.

11. Kolar OJ, Ross AT, Herman JT: Serum and cerebrospinal fluid immunoglobulins in multiple sclerosis. *Neurology* **20**:1052-1061, 1970.

12. Dencker SJ, Kolar O: The cerebrospinal fluid γ-globulin profile in subacute sclerosing leucoencephalitis. *Acta Neurol Scand* **41**(suppl 13):135-140, 1965.

13. Meulemans O: Determination of total protein in spinal fluid with sulfosalicylic acid and trichloroacetic acid. *Clin Chim Acta* **5**:757-761, 1960.

14. Whitaker JN, Lemmi H: A rapid method for the concentration of cerebrospinal fluid proteins prior to paper electrophoresis. *Tech Bull Reg Med Tech* **36**:91-94, 1966.

15. Mancini G, Vaerman JP, Carbonara AO, et al: A single-radial-diffusion method for the immunological quantitation of proteins, in Peeters H (ed): *Protides of the Biological Fluids: Proceedings of the XI Colloquium.* Amsterdam, Elsevier Publishing Co, 1963, pp 370-373.

16. Uyeda CT, Gerstl B, Eng LF, et al: Serum immunoglobulins in multiple sclerosis patients. *Proc Soc Exp Biol Med* **131**:1138, 1969.

17. McAlpine D, Lumsden CE, Acheson ED: *Multiple Sclerosis: A Reappraisal.* Edinburgh, Scotland, E & S Livingstone Ltd, 1968, pp 94-119.

18. Takase S, Yoshida M: Quantitative determination of immunoglobulins in CSF. *Tohoku J Exp Med* **98**:189-198, 1969.

19. Laterre EC, Heremans JF, Carbonara AD: Immunological comparison of some proteins found in CSF, urine and extracts from brain and kidney. *Clin Chim Acta* **10**:197-209, 1969.

20. Van Welsum RA, Van Der Helm HJ: The protein composition of the cerebrospinal fluid in acute necrotizing encephalitis: An agar gel electrophoretic and immunoelectrophoretic study. *Neurology* **20**:996-1001, 1970.

21. Hunter R, Jones M, Malleson A: Abnormal cerebrospinal fluid total protein and gammaglobulin levels in 256 patients admitted to psychiatric unit. *J Neurol Sci* **9**:11-38, 1969.

22. Tourtellotte WW, Parker JA: Multiple sclerosis: Brain immunoglobulin-G and albumin. *Nature* **214**:683-686, 1967.

23. Kolar O, Dencker SJ, Obrucnik M, et al: Zur bedeutung der gamma G-globulinfraktion im hirngewebe bei der subakuten sklerotisierenden leukoencephalitis. *Deutsch Z Nervenheilk* **188**:222-233, 1966.

24. Gerstl B, Uyeda CT, Eng LE, et al: Soluble proteins in normal and diseased human brains. *Neurology* **19**:1019-1026, 1969.

25. Bourdillon RB, Fischer-Williams M, Smith HV, et al: The entry of radiosodium and of bromide into human cerebrospinal fluid. *J Neurol Neurosurg Psychiat* **20**:79-97, 1957.

26. Haerer AF, Tourtellotte WW, Richard KA, et al: A study of the blood-cerebrospinal fluid-brain barrier in multiple sclerosis: I. Blood-cerebrospinal fluid barrier to sodium bromide. *Neurology* **14**:345-354, 1964.

27. Dau PC, Peterson RDA: Transformation of lymphocytes from patients with multiple sclerosis: Use of an encephalitogen of human origin, with a report of a trial of immunosuppressive therapy in multiple sclerosis. *Arch Neurol* **23**:32-40, 1970.

28. Fowler I, Morris CE, Whitley T: Lymphocyte transformation in multiple sclerosis induced by cerebrospinal fluid. *New Eng J Med* **275**:1041-1044, 1966.

29. Brody JA, Harlem MM, Kurtzke JF, et al: Unsuccessful attempt to induce transformation by cerebrospinal fluid in cultured lymphocytes from patients with multiple sclerosis. *New Eng J Med* **279**:202-204, 1968.

30. Carnegie PR: Properties, structure and possible neuroreceptor role of the encephalitogenic protein of human brain. *Nature* **229**:25-28, 1971.

120

Immunoglobulins in Multiple Sclerosis and Infections of the Nervous System

Hans Link, MD, and Ragnar Müller, MD

CONSIDERABLE research has been carried out in order to find abnormalities in the cerebrospinal fluid (CSF) characteristic of multiple sclerosis (MS). Hitherto the most useful biochemical diagnostic tool has been the quantitation of immunoglobulin G (IgG) in CSF by means of immunoprecipitation[1-3] and more recently by means of electroimmunodiffusion[4] and radial immunodiffusion.[5] Early in these studies it became clear that the determination of the relative CSF immunoglobulin concentrations (ie, expressed in percent of total CSF protein concentration) rather than of the absolute CSF immunoglobulin concentrations (ie, expressed in mg/100 ml) is of greater significance in demonstrating changes in the concentrations of the individual immunoglobulins. In this way relative CSF-IgG concentrations have been shown to be increased in 80% of patients with MS.[2] Serum IgG concentrations have, however, not been shown to increase significantly in this disorder.[2,6,7]

Determination of the relative CSF-IgG concentration by any of the techniques mentioned are now used routinely in most laboratories when a diagnosis of MS is considered. These techniques have replaced the more inaccurate and insensitive procedures, such as the colloidal curves and the quantitation of the gamma globulin fraction after electrophoresis on different supporting media.

More recently, other CSF-IgG abnormalities have been found to occur in MS. By immunoelectrophoresis, abnormalities of the IgG precipitation line have been demonstrated.[8,9] By agar gel electrophoresis, IgG of

MS-CSF has been shown to behave as electrophoretically homogeneous, and it appears in the form of two or more discrete bands.[10] The value of agar gel electrophoresis of CSF for the diagnosis of MS and the superiority of agar gel over other supporting media for the demonstration of CSF immunoglobulin abnormalities has been established.[10,11] By quantitation of immunoglobulin light chains of types kappa and lambda, it has been found that MS-CSF may contain IgG with an abnormal light chain distribution, most commonly with an increase in the ratio of kappa: lambda light chains.[12] The frequency of occurrence of an abnormal kappa:lambda ratio in MS or in any other neurological disorder is, however, unknown.

The purpose of this paper is to determine and to compare the frequencies of occurrence of the above summarized abnormalities in MS-CSF and in the CSF of patients with other neurological disorders. An attempt is made to ascertain which method of investigation of CSF is the most useful for establishing the diagnosis of MS. Among the other neurological disorders, special attention is paid to infections of the nervous system because of the similarities among findings in this group of disorders and in MS. Such similarities include mononuclear pleocytosis, increased relative CSF-IgG concentrations,[2] and the appearance of discrete bands in the gamma region on agar gel electrophoresis.[11]

In addition, the purpose of the present communication is to evaluate if there exists in MS a correlation between the occurrence of some of the above mentioned abnormalities in the CSF and of different clinical factors.

Materials

Cerebrospinal fluid and serum samples were obtained from the following four groups:

Group 1.—Thirty "healthy controls" (ie, volunteers or persons with minor psychoneurotic disorders).[10] In order to qualify as a healthy control, the volunteer or patient must have had a CSF white blood cell count of 5/cu mm or less and a total CSF protein concentration less than 46 mg/100 ml.

Group 2.—Sixty-four consecutive patients with MS, diagnosed according to clinical criteria[13] and without taking into account the CSF findings. The following three criteria must have

been met in order to permit a diagnosis of MS: age of onset between 15 and 45 years; signs indicative of damage to at least two different parts of the central nervous system (CNS); and a course with at least two exacerbations and one remission. In addition, no signs of other disorders were present in any of the MS patients. Four of the patients were on small doses of adenocorticotropic hormone at the time of lumbar puncture.

The MS patients were divided into two groups regarding disability: (a) 43 patients without disability at all or with only slight disability, ie, patients who were able to manage themselves in every respect and who had symptoms and signs which not at all or only slightly influenced professional and social life. (b) 21 patients with moderate or great disability, ie, patients who were depending to a varying degree on assistance and whose professional and social life was influenced to a moderate or considerable degree.

Group 3.—Thirty-nine patients with infectious disorders of the nervous system, including ten consecutive patients with neurosyphilis. Only one of the neurosyphilis patients (case 30, Table 9) had not been treated with penicillin prior to puncture.

Group 4.—Eighty-one patients with various neurological disorders other than MS and infections of the nervous system. The specific diagnoses included in this group were as follows: tumor of the CNS (23); degenerative nervous disease (14); polyneuropathy (13); senile dementia (9); epilepsy (9); cerebrovascular disease (4); rizopathy (4); paralysis agitans (3); cerebral concussion (2).

The sex and age distribution of the cases in the different patient groups are given in Table 1.

After differential cell counting, centrifugation, and determination of the total CSF protein concentration, 1 ml of each CSF specimen was stored at −20 C, while the remainder was concentrated by ultrafiltration in collodion bags at 4 C, to a protein concentration of 8.0 gm/100 ml, and then stored at −20 C along with the corresponding serum specimen.[10]

Antisera.—Rabbit antisera against human CSF and serum, and against human serum IgG, were prepared as described.[10] Specific antisera against light chains of type kappa and lambda, respectively, were prepared as described.[12]

A rabbit antiserum against heavy chains from normal human serum IgG was prepared as previously described.[10] This antiserum was absorbed with normal human light chains. No cross reaction was obtained with light chains in immunodiffusions.

Specific rabbit antisera against human serum

immunoglobulin A (IgA) and immunoglobulin M (IgM) were obtained from commercial sources.

Methods

Single Radial Immunodiffusion.—This was performed according to Mancini et al as described previously[10] for quantitation of IgG, IgA, and IgM, and of light chains of types kappa and lambda. Suitably diluted antiserum was preheated to 56 C and maintained at that temperature for 30 minutes. The antiserum was then incorporated into a 3% agar (Difco Special Agar Noble) in pH 8.0 buffer containing 0.03M sodium phosphate and 0.1M sodium chloride. Immunodiffusion was allowed to proceed at room temperature for 48 hours in a chamber with high humidity.

Serial dilutions of pooled normal blood donor serum were used as standards. This pool comprised equal amounts of serum from 30 healthy Swedish blood donors. Immediately after receipt, the blood donor serum was divided into samples of 0.2 ml which were stored at −20 C until use. None of the samples used as standards had been refrozen. The same pool of blood donor serum was used as the standard for all of the quantitations carried out in the present investigation. The standard serum was assigned the following immunoglobulin concentrations: IgG, 1.000 mg/100 ml; IgA, 200 mg/100 ml; and IgM, 75 mg/100 ml. These values were taken from the literature and refer to Swedish blood donors.[14] The lower limit for detection of IgA was 0.20 mg/100 ml, and for IgM this limit was 0.25 mg/100 ml. The kappa:lambda ratio in the pooled normal blood donor serum standard was arbitrarily assigned a value of 1.0.[12]

The quantitations on the CSF and serum samples were carried out from one week to six months after lumbar puncture. Thus, only previously frozen samples were investigated. Mostly, freezing and thawing of the samples was performed only once before the quantitations.

Agar Gel Electrophoresis.—This procedure was carried out on microscope slides according to Wieme under conditions described earlier[10] but with the following modifications: 1 µl of CSF concentrated to a total protein concentration of about 8.0 gm/100 ml was deposited per millimeter of the trough. Electrophoresis was run at 10 to 12 C for 28 minutes at 220 v (rather than 25 minutes at 200 v), and the staining solution contained Amido black 10 B, 0.5 gm; mercuric chloride, 5.0 gm; glacial acetic acid, 5 ml; and distilled water up to 1,000 ml (rather than 100 ml). The electrophoresis was performed within 24 hours after lumbar puncture

on previously unfrozen samples of concentrated CSF and of serum. The slides were inspected and the occurrence of two or more discrete bands in the gamma region in position between beta-trace protein and gamma-trace protein was considered to be pathologic.[10]

Immunoelectrophoresis.—Previously frozen samples of concentrated CSF and serum were used according to a modified Scheidegger micromethod as previously described in detail.[10] The same batch of rabbit antiserum against human serum was used in all immunoelectrophoresis procedures.

Protein Concentration.—Determinations were made by a modified Lowry method.[15]

Results

The results obtained in the present investigation are, for purposes of clarity, best presented in terms of the controls and the three patient groups studied. The ranges and mean values for the total CSF protein concentration for IgG, IgA, and IgM concentrations and for the kappa:lambda ratios in both CSF and serum found in each of the four groups are given in Table 2.

Healthy Controls.—The upper normal limit was defined as the mean value of the controls plus 2 standard deviations. Since, however, the CSF-IgA concentration was not measurable (ie, was less than 0.20 mg/100 ml) in 14 of the controls, no mean value and standard deviation for IgA are given in the Table. The highest CSF-IgA concentration found among the control cases (0.6 mg/100 ml, which corresponded to a relative CSF-IgA concentration of 1.9%) was used as the upper normal concentration limit for CSF-IgA. CSF-IgM was not measurable (less than 0.25 mg/100 ml) in any of the control samples analyzed.

Multiple Sclerosis.—The frequencies of occurrence of the various abnormal findings in the CSF samples from the 64 MS patients are given in Table 3. More than five mononuclear leukocytes per cubic millimeter were found in 50% of the cases. The total protein concentration was increased above normal (above 45 mg/100 ml) in 66% of the cases. The total protein concentration was above 60 mg/100 ml in 26 of the cases (41%). In 73% of the 64 MS cases studied, the relative CSF-IgG concentration exceeded the upper normal value of 10.5% of the total CSF protein concentration. The CSF-IgA concentration was not measurable (less than 0.20 mg/100 ml) in 14 of the MS cases. Increased relative CSF-IgA concentrations (ie, those above 1.9% of the total CSF protein) were found in 9% of the cases. No CSF-IgM concentrations above 0.25 mg/100 ml were found in any of the 64 MS cases studied. Elevated kappa:lambda ratios (greater than 1.7) were found in 53% of the MS-CSF samples analyzed. A ratio below the lower normal value (ie, 0.5) was found in one case.

Two abnormalities in the appearance of the IgG precipitation line were detected when immunoelectrophoresis was carried out on the CSF and serum samples from the MS patient group. An extra IgG precipitation line in the cathode (Fig 1, *upper arrow*) as well as a doubling of the IgG precipitation line (Fig 1, *lower arrow*) were found at the same time in eight of the 62 MS-CSF samples investigated (13%). In 11 of the cases (18%) only a cathodic extra IgG line was found, and in eight cases (13%) only a doubling of the IgG precipitation line was observed. Thus, in 44% of the MS-CSF samples analyzed, abnormalities of the IgG precipitation line were detected. The corresponding serum patterns appeared normal in all of the 64 MS cases as did the patterns of the 30 control CSF and serum samples studied (Fig 1).

Neither abnormality was demonstrable when immunoelectrophoresis was carried out with an antiserum against heavy chains, nor after absorption of the antiserum against human serum with light chains (Fig 1). This indicates that both abnormalities are due to light chain antigenic determinants.

The kappa:lambda ratio was abnormally high in all of those cases in which immunoelectrophoresis of CSF showed a doubling of the IgG precipitation line. In the 11 cases in which only a cathodic extra arc was observed, the kappa:lambda ratio was abnormally high in four of the cases.

At least two discrete IgG bands (Fig 2, *B* and *C*) were demonstrated on agar gel electrophoresis in 60 of the 64 MS-CSF samples investigated (94%), whereas the serum patterns were found to be normal in all of these cases. No discrete IgG bands were found in any of the 30 control CSF or serum samples.

In three of the four MS-CSF samples which showed normal agar gel electrophoresis patterns, all of the other CSF investigations were normal, while the fourth patient had an increased total CSF protein concentration as the only abnormality.

In Table 4 the 64 MS cases have been divided into two groups, one with normal relative CSF-IgG concentrations and the other with increased relative CSF-IgG concentrations. Among the 47 cases with increased relative CSF-IgG concentrations, discrete IgG bands were found on CSF agar gel electrophoresis in all cases. Among the 17 cases with normal relative CSF-IgG concentrations, discrete IgG bands were found in only 77% of the cases. Mononuclear pleocytosis and an abnormal kappa:lambda ratio were also found more often among the cases with increased relative CSF-IgG concentrations than among the cases with normal relative CSF-IgG concentrations.

Increased serum IgG concentrations (greater than 1.7 gm/100 ml) were found in three of the 64 MS cases studied, and increased serum IgM concentrations (greater than 170 mg/100 ml) in four. The three cases with increased serum IgG concentrations also had abnormally high relative CSF-IgG concentrations. No abnormally high serum IgA concentrations were found in any of the 64 MS cases (Table 2).

The frequencies of occurrence of increased number of mononuclear leukocytes, increased total CSF protein concentration, increased relative CSF-IgG concentration, and abnormally high kappa:lambda ratio found among the MS-CSF samples are given in relation to various clinical factors in Tables 5 to 8. A difference between the percentages was considered significant when $P < 0.05$.

The patient group with the highest age at the time of lumbar puncture (Table 5) also presented a significantly lower frequency of occurrence of mononuclear pleocytosis and a significantly higher frequency of occurrence of abnormally high total CSF protein concentration than younger patient groups.

In the patient group with the longest duration of disease (Table 6), the frequency of occurrence of mononuclear pleocytosis and of abnormally high kappa:lambda ratio was significantly lower than in the two patient groups taken together with a shorter duration.

No significant differences were noticed between the frequencies of occurrence of the different abnormal CSF findings when related to the time interval between the last exacerbation of symptoms and lumbar puncture (Table 7).

When comparing the two patient groups according to a different disability rate, there was a significantly lower frequency of occurrence of mononuclear pleocytosis and a significantly higher frequency of occurrence of elevated total CSF protein concentration in the patient group with moderate or severe disability (Table 8).

Infectious Disorders of the Nervous System.—The frequencies of occurrence of the different abnormalities found among the CSF samples from the 39 patients with infectious disorders of the nervous system are given in Table 3, and the details of the individual cases are presented for reference purposes in Table 9.

It is evident from the data presented in these tables that increased relative CSF immunoglobulin concentrations frequently occur in infections of the nervous system. Increased relative CSF-IgG concentrations were found in 12 of the 33 CSF samples investigated. These 12 cases included four of the eight patients with neurosyphilis and the two patients with encephalitis due to herpes simplex infection.

Increased relative CSF-IgA concentrations were found in nine of the 33 CSF samples investigated. These nine cases included all five of the patients with herpes zoster in whom lumbar puncture was performed within 36 days after the onset of the disease, one of the two patients with encephalitis due to herpes simplex infection and one of the eight patients with neurosyphilis whose CSF samples were available for analysis.

Two of the five patients with herpes zoster in whom lumbar puncture was performed within 36 days after the onset of the disease had shown acute manifestations of the disease without any clinical signs of CNS involvement. In the two cases of herpes zoster which had occurred two years prior to lumbar puncture and which also showed no

signs of CNS involvement, relative CSF-IgA concentrations were within normal limits, the only CSF abnormality observed being an increased total CSF protein concentration in one of the two cases. These findings indicate that in herpes zoster increased relative CSF-IgA concentrations may occur in the earlier stages of the disease.

As no absolute CSF-IgM concentrations above 0.25 mg/100 ml were found in any of the control cases studied, only relative CSF-IgM concentrations above 1.2% of the total CSF protein concentration are suggested as being abnormally increased. (This suggestion is based on the assumption that 0.25 mg/100 ml can be taken as the highest normal absolute CSF-IgM concentration and on the assumption that 21 mg/100 ml can be taken as the lowest total CSF protein concentration, as was found among the 30 control CSF samples studied in this investigation.) Increased relative CSF-IgM concentrations were found only in two of the patients with aseptic meningitis and in the one case of untreated neurosyphilis.

The serum IgG, IgA, and IgM concentrations for 23 of the cases in the group of patients with infectious disorders of the nervous system were determined and were found to be within normal limits in all cases with the exception of slightly increased IgG concentrations in two cases (case 25 with herpes zoster and normal relative CSF-IgG concentration and case 30 with neurosyphilis and slightly increased relative CSF-IgG concentration, Table 9) and of increased IgM concentrations in two cases (case 14 with chronic aseptic meningitis and case 32 with neurosyphilis). In both of these cases, the relative CSF-IgM concentrations were, however, less than 1.2% of the respective total CSF protein concentrations.

In contrast to the findings among the 64 MS patients, no abnormal CSF kappa: lambda ratios were found among the cases with infectious disorders of the nervous system. One patient with mumps meningitis (case 5, Table 9) had a slightly increased (1.8) serum kappa:lambda ratio.

An extra IgG precipitation line in the cathode and a doubling of the IgG precipitation line were found in CSF in one case of mumps meningitis and in one case of acute aseptic meningitis, while only an extra IgG

125

precipitation line in the cathode was found in each of the five additional samples. Neither abnormality was found in the serum from any of the 33 patients in whom immunoelectrophoresis was carried out.

At least two discrete bands in the gamma region on CSF agar gel electrophoresis were found in 39% of the cases, namely in one case of acute and in one case of chronic aseptic meningitis, in both cases of encephalitis due to herpes simplex infection, in the two cases of herpes zoster with CNS involvement, in two of the three cases of toxoplasmosis, and in all but three of the cases of neurosyphilis. A faint band in the serum gamma region corresponding to one of the discrete gamma bands observed in the CSF was demonstrable in one case of herpes zoster encephalitis and in one case of toxoplasmosis. The serum agar gel electrophoresis patterns were normal in all of the other cases.

Other Neurological Disorders.—The frequencies of occurrence of the different CSF abnormalities found in the patient group consisting of 81 cases with neurological disorders other than MS and infectious disorders of the nervous system are also given in Table 3. Increased relative CSF-IgG concentrations were found in 13 of the cases (16%). The increase was only slight (10.6% to 14.5% of the total CSF protein concentrations) in ten of the 13 cases. Six of these ten cases had tumors within the CNS. The total CSF protein concentration was at least 85 mg/100 ml in eight of the ten cases with slightly increased relative CSF-IgG concentrations.

In the remaining three of the 13 cases with increased relative CSF-IgG concentrations, the degree of increase was quite marked. These three cases included one case of medullary tumor, one case of dementia, and one case of multiple myeloma with medullary compression in which the relative CSF-IgG concentrations were found to be 17.9%, 26.5%, and 47.0%, respectively. The total CSF protein concentrations in these three cases were 577, 23, and 139 mg/100 ml, respectively.

The serum IgG concentrations were found to be increased (range of 1.8 to 4.0 gm/100 ml) in six of the 81 cases investigated. Five of these six cases had normal relative CSF-

IgG concentrations, and one case, the patient with multiple myeloma, showed a marked increase in the relative CSF-IgG concentration (47.0%).

Increased relative CSF-IgA concentrations (range of 2.0% to 5.8% of the respective total CSF protein concentrations) were found in 11 of the 81 cases studied (14%). Nine of these 11 patients had tumors within the CNS, and each was found to have a total CSF protein concentration above 100 mg/100 ml. The remaining two patients had cerebellar degeneration, probably due to alcoholic abuse, and cerebrovascular disease, respectively, and the total CSF protein concentrations were 41 and 62 mg/100 ml. The serum IgA concentrations were within normal limits in all the 11 cases with increased relative CSF-IgA concentrations.

Increased relative CSF-IgM concentrations were found in five of the 81 cases (6%). Three of these five patients had tumors within the CNS and increased total CSF protein concentrations, while the remaining two patients had epilepsy and a degenerative nervous disease, respectively, and normal total CSF protein concentrations. The serum IgM concentrations were normal in all of the five cases with increased relative CSF-IgM concentrations.

Increased CSF kappa:lambda ratios were found in two of the 81 cases (3%). These two cases included one case of multiple myeloma with medullary compression and one case of polyneuropathy in which the kappa:lambda ratios were found to be 17.3 and 1.9, respectively. No abnormally low CSF kappa:lambda ratios were found. The serum kappa:lambda ratio was increased (10.0) in the one case of multiple myeloma and normal in the remaining 80 cases.

Cerebrospinal fluid and serum samples from only 46 of the 81 cases were studied by immunoelectrophoresis due to lack of sufficient amounts of material. Abnormalities on immunoelectrophoresis were found in seven of the 46 CSF samples investigated (15%). An extra IgG precipitation line in the cathode and a doubling of the IgG precipitation line were found in two cases, including the patient with polyneuropathy and an increased CSF kappa:lambda ratio, while only an extra IgG precipitation line in the cathode was found in each of the remaining five cases. The diagnoses in these five cases were quite varied. Neither abnormality was found on investigation of the serum samples from any of these 46 cases.

At least two discrete bands in the gamma region on agar gel electrophoresis of CSF samples from this patient group were found in one of the two cases of syringomyelia and in one case of polyneuropathy. The patient with polyneuropathy was 60 years old and was also found to have an increased CSF kappa:lambda ratio (1.9) as well as an extra precipitation line in the cathode and a doubling of the IgG precipitation line on CSF immunoelectrophoresis. Only one discrete band was demonstrable in the gamma region in both the CSF and the serum of the patient with multiple myeloma. Serum agar gel electrophoresis patterns were found to be normal in all the other cases.

Comment

Immunoglobulin Concentrations.—Several immunochemical (eg, immunoprecipitation, radial immunodiffusion, and electroimmunodiffusion) analytic methods are presently available for the determination of immunoglobulin concentrations in unconcentrated CSF and in serum. Differences in the sensitivities of these methods must be considered in the evaluation of the results; eg, commercially available immunodiffusion plates can probably not be used for the quantitation of individual CSF immunoglobulins without previous concentration of the fluid,[5] thus introducing a considerable error to the estimations.

The absolute CSF-IgG concentrations found among the control samples in the present investigation agree well with the normal values obtained by Kabat et al,[1] when using immunoprecipitation, and with those obtained by Hartley et al,[4] when using electroimmunodiffusion. The relative CSF-IgG concentrations determined from the control samples investigated in the present work also agree reasonably well with the normal values previously reported by Kabat et al.[1]

Normal CSF-IgA concentrations have previously been determined only for concentrated CSF samples. Hartley et al,[4] when using electroimmunodiffusion, found a range of 0.10 to 0.25 mg/100 ml with an average of 0.17 mg/100 ml in their study of ten normal CSF samples, while Bauer and Gottesleben,[5] when using radial immunodiffusion, found a mean value of 0.226 mg/100 ml in 48 normal controls. The last group of investigators, however, did not give any data about their criteria for "normal."

The absolute CSF-IgA concentrations determined in the present investigation of 30 unconcentrated control CSF samples were found to be somewhat higher than the normal values reported in the above studies. The differences may be due to protein aggregation and losses during the concentration procedures used in the previous investigations.

No normal CSF-IgM concentrations have hitherto been established. The finding in the present investigation of absolute CSF-IgM concentrations below 0.25 mg/100 ml is consistent with earlier reports that it is not possible to demonstrate IgM in unconcentrated normal CSF with the methods available at present.[4]

Among the MS cases studied in the present investigation, the frequency of occurrence (73% of cases) of increased relative CSF-IgG concentrations (greater than 10.5% of the total CSF protein concentration) agrees reasonably well with the frequencies reported by Kabat et al[2] (80% when using immunoprecipitation) and by Yahr et el[3] (66.5% when using immunoprecipitation), but it is higher than the frequencies reported by Schneck and Claman[16] (56% when using electroimmunodiffusion) and by Riddoch and Thompson[17] (62% when using radial immunodiffusion). The discrepancies may, among other things, be due to differences in the selection of the cases studied, as the relative CSF-IgG concentration may be influenced by different clinical factors (see below).

CSF-IgA concentrations in MS-CSF have previously been investigated by two groups of investigators. Schneck and Claman[16] determined the absolute IgA concentrations in 48 unconcentrated MS-CSF samples by means of electroimmunodiffusion and found concentrations above 0.4 mg/100 ml in 12 of the samples. Bauer and Gottesleben[5] when using radial immunodiffusion found increased absolute IgA concentrations in 20 out of 55 MS-CSF samples investigated. These samples were, however, investigated after previous concentration as were the controls (see above). Both groups of investigators did not report the relative CSF-IgA concentrations.

A finding of increased absolute CSF-IgA concentration may be expected to occur, among others, in cases with blood-CSF barrier damage and increased total CSF protein concentration, the increase of the CSF-IgA concentration being proportional to the increase of the total CSF protein concentration.[18] Therefore, the finding of an increased absolute CSF-IgA concentration probably does not give information beyond that obtained by determination of the total CSF protein concentration. Only a finding of increased relative CSF-IgA concentration may provide some basis for, eg, the hypothesis of synthesis of the protein within the CNS.

Increased relative CSF-IgA concentrations were found in only 9% of the 64 MS-CSF samples studied. This frequency of occurrence is lower than the frequency found among the CSF samples from the patients with infectious disorders of the nervous system (27%) and also somewhat lower than the frequency found among the CSF samples from the patients with other neurological disorders (14%).

Although the in vitro synthesis of IgA has previously been demonstrated using lymphocytes from the CSF of one patient with MS,[19] the low frequency of occurrence of increased relative CSF-IgA concentrations among the MS patients studied indicates that synthesis of IgA within the CNS probably does not occur to an extent capable of elevating relative CSF-IgA concentrations above normal limits in this disorder.

The finding of absolute CSF-IgM concentrations below 0.25 mg/100 ml in all of the 64 MS cases studied is consistent with the recent finding by Schneck and Claman[16] who used electroimmunodiffusion and found that increased absolute CSF-IgM concentrations rarely occur in this disorder.

The serum immunoglobulin concentrations found among the 30 controls agree fairly well with the normal serum immunoglobulin concentrations reported by Norberg.[14] The finding of normal serum IgG concentrations in all but three of the 64 MS-CSF samples is in accordance with the findings by Kabat et al[2] and by Uyeda et al[7] that serum IgG concentrations are usually normal in this disorder, even in cases where increased relative CSF-IgG concentrations are found.

Significantly increased serum IgA concentrations and significantly decreased serum IgM concentrations have recently been reported by Uyeda et al[7] in their investigation of 57 MS cases. These findings are contrary to the findings in the present investigation. No explanation can be given at present for this discrepancy.

Increased relative CSF concentrations of IgG, IgA, and IgM were found in a variety of infections of the nervous system (Table 9). There appears to be no simultaneous increase in the CSF concentrations of the three immunoglobulins but rather a selective increase in one or two of them. Of special interest is the finding of increased relative CSF-IgA concentration in all five cases with herpes zoster where the CSF was obtained within 36 days after the beginning of the disease. However, the cases presented in Table 9 are too heterogeneous, and the number of cases of any single disorder is too small to allow any conclusions to be drawn in regard to possible patterns of alterations in CSF immunoglobulin concentrations during the course of any given infection.

Increased relative CSF-IgG concentrations were also found in 16% of the 81 cases with neurological disorders other than MS or infectious disorders of the nervous system. This frequency of occurrence agrees reasonably well with the frequencies reported by Kabat et al[2] (22%), by Schneck and Claman[16] (12%), and by Riddoch and Thompson[17] (14%).

Increased relative CSF-IgG concentrations were found significantly more often in MS than in infectious disorders of the nervous system ($0.01 < P < 0.02$) and in the group of patients with other neurological disorders ($P < 0.01$). The difference between the frequency of occurrence of increased relative CSF-IgG concentrations in infectious disorders and in disorders other than MS and infections was not significant.

No significant differences were found in the frequencies of occurrence of elevated relative CSF-IgA concentrations in the three groups of patients investigated.

At present, two explanations seem most tenable for the finding of increased relative immunoglobulin concentrations in neurological disorders. These are (1) synthesis within the CNS, and (2) migration from serum to CSF due to blood-CSF barrier damage.

The occurrence of increased relative CSF-IgG concentrations in MS has been attributed by Kabat et al[2] to the synthesis of IgG within the CNS. This hypothesis seems to have been proven by the finding that in both patients with MS and in those with neurosyphilis, the specific activity of ^{131}I-labeled IgG injected intravenously remains considerably lower in CSF than in serum.[20] The serum immunoglobulin concentrations may well influence CSF immunoglobulin concentrations, but neither the fre-

quency of occurrence (73% of cases) of increased relative CSF-IgG concentrations found among the MS patients nor the frequency (36% of cases) found among the patients with infectious disorders of the nervous system can be accounted for by concomitant increases in the serum IgG concentrations in these patients. Indeed, abnormally high serum IgG concentrations were found in only three of the 64 MS cases and in only two of the 23 samples from cases with infectious disorders of the nervous system in which quantitation was carried out.

The cause of increased relative CSF-IgG concentrations reported in cases with neurological disorders other than MS or infectious disorders of the nervous system is not known. An increased serum IgG concentration was found in only one of the 13 cases observed in the present investigation with

Table 1.—Sex and Age Distribution

Age (yr)	Controls (n=30)		MS (n=64)		Infectious Disorders of the Nervous System (n=39)		Other Neurological Disorders (n=81)	
	Men	Women	Men	Women	Men	Women	Men	Women
≦10	...	...	...	...	2	4	...	...
11-20	...	1	...	1	1	4	4	1
21-30	3	9	9	11	4	1	7	4
31-40	2	5	6	13	4	2	6	5
41-50	2	4	7	7	...	2	10	8
51-60	1	1	4	6	4	...	25	11
>60	2	...	...	...	4	7	...	...

Table 2.—Ranges and Mean Values for Total CSF Protein Concentration, Immunoglobulin

	Total CSF Protein Concentration (mg/100 ml)	IgG Concentration		
		CSF		Serum (mg/100 ml)
		mg/100 ml	%*	
Controls (n=30) Range	21-45	0.8-3.5	2.8-10.6	0.5-1.6
Mean value	33	2.2	6.1	1.1
Standard deviation	6	0.7	2.2	0.3
Multiple sclerosis (n=64) Range	26-101	1.5-27.0	4.1-42.0	0.7-1.9
Mean value	55	8.4	15.0	1.2
Infectious disorders of the nervous system (n=39) Range	23-1.180	1.3-64.4	3.7-29.5	0.9-1.8
Mean value	110	9.8 (n=33)	10.2 (n=33)	1.3 (n=23)
Other neurological disorders (n=81) Range	19-577	1.3-103.0	2.3-47.0	0.6-4.0
Mean value	90	9.7	8.5	1.3

* Percent of total CSF protein concentration.
† For definition see introduction.

increased relative CSF-IgG concentrations —a patient with multiple myeloma—and therefore cannot account for the abnormality in the 12 remaining cases. Increases in the total CSF protein concentration may, if derived from migration of serum proteins into the CSF due to blood-CSF barrier damage, bring the relative CSF-IgG concentrations closer to the IgG percentages found in the serum samples, since the percentage of IgG relative to the total protein concentration is usually higher in serum than it is in CSF. As a matter of fact, nine of the 12 remaining cases with increased relative CSF-IgG concentrations had total CSF protein concentrations above 85 mg/100 ml. These increases in the total CSF protein concentrations may, at least in part, be contributing to the increased relative CSF-IgG concentrations, and they may also play a role in those cases in which the relative CSF-IgA and CSF-IgM concentrations are found to be increased. However, an intrathecal synthesis of these three immunoglobulins is not in any way excluded.

Kappa:Lambda Ratio.—The kappa:lambda ratios of the control CSF and serum samples agree well with previously determined ratios obtained when another normal blood donor serum standard was used.[12] The choice of pooled blood donor serum as the standard for quantitation of kappa and lambda light chain antigenic determinants seemed to be appropriate as this method had previously been used effectively for the quantitation of IgG, IgA, and IgM in body fluids.[14]

Increased kappa:lambda ratios in MS have previously been demonstrated in six of 14 CSF samples from patients whose corresponding serum ratios were all found to be within normal limits.[12] These earlier results are corroborated by the finding in the present investigation of increased CSF kappa:lambda ratios in 53% of the 64 MS-CSF samples studied, all of which were found to have normal serum ratios.

Surprisingly, increased kappa:lambda ratios were not found in any of the CSF samples from patients with infectious disorders of the nervous system, despite the frequent finding of other CSF immunoglobulin abnormalities in these cases. In the cases with neurological disorders other than MS and infectious disorders, and when excluding the patient with multiple myeloma, an increased kappa:lambda ratio was found in only one out of the 80 CSF samples investigated, while the corresponding serum kappa:lambda ratios were normal in all.

The low frequency of occurrence of abnormal CSF kappa:lambda ratios in the patients with neurological disorders other than MS suggests that determination of the distribution of immunoglobulin light chain de-

Concentrations, and Kappa:Lambda Ratios in the Controls and in the Three Patient Groups

| IgA Concentration | | | IgM Concentration | | | Kappa: Lambda Ratio† | |
| CSF | | Serum | CSF | | Serum | | |
mg/100 ml	%*	(mg/100 ml)	mg/100 ml	%*	(mg/100 ml)	CSF	Serum
≤0.2-0.6	0.4-1.9 (n=16)	60-520	...	...	25-190	0.5-1.7	0.4-1.8
...	...	260	...	...	90	1.1	1.1
...	...	120	...	...	40	0.3	0.3
≤0.2-1.6	0.2-3.7 (n=50)	60-440	...	...	25-330	0.4-8.7	0.7-1.5
...	...	180	...	...	101	2.4	1.1
≤0.2-21.6 (n=33)	0.3-4.9 (n=29)	180-470	≤0.25-5.4 (n=33)	0.2-2.7 (n=12)	50-258	0.3-1.7	0.5-1.8
...	...	318 (n=23)	...	...	112 (n=23)	0.9 (n=37)	1.1 (n=26)
≤0.2-30.5	0.3-5.8 (n=63)	60-700	≤0.25-7.8	0.2-5.0 (n=23)	25-305	0.5-17.3	0.6-10.0
...	...	256	...	...	87	1.1	1.2

Table 3.—Frequencies of Abnormal CSF Findings

Abnormal CSF Findings	% in MS (n = 64)	% in Infectious Disorders of the Nervous System (n = 39)	% in Other Neurological Disorders (n = 81)
Mononuclear leukocytes >5/cu mm	50	66 (n = 35)	17
Increased total protein concentration (>45 mg/100 ml)	66	64	59
Increased relative IgG concentration (>10.5% of total CSF protein concentration)	73	36 (n = 33)	16
Increased relative IgA concentration (>1.9% of total CSF protein concentration)	9	27 (n=33)	14
Increased relative IgM concentration (>1.2% of total CSF protein concentration)	0	9 (n = 33)	6
Increased kappa: lambda ratio (>1.7)	53	0 (n = 37)	3
Abnormalities of the IgG precipitation line on immunoelectrophoresis	44 (n = 62)	21 (n = 33)	15 (n = 46)
Abnormal bands on agar gel electrophoresis	94	39	3 (n = 75)*

* One abnormal band was visible in the gamma region of CSF and serum from one additional patient who suffered of multiple myeloma.

Table 4.—CSF-IgG Concentration in Relation to Other Abnormal CSF Findings in 64 Patients With Multiple Sclerosis

	Total Protein Concentration >45 mg/100 ml (%)	Mononuclear Leukocytes >5/cu mm (%)	Abnormal Bands on Agar Gel Electrophoresis (%)	Abnormalities of the IgG Precipitation Line on Immunoelectrophoresis (%)	Kappa: Lambda Ratio >1.7 (%)
CSF-IgG ≤10.5% (n = 17)	10 (59)	5 (29)	13 (77)	5/15 (33)	3 (18)
CSF-IgG >10.5% (n = 47)	32 (68)	27 (58)	47 (100)	22/47 (47)	31 (66)

Table 5.—Frequencies of Abnormal MS-CSF Findings in Relation to Age at Lumbar Puncture

Age (yr)	Mononuclear Leukocytes >5/cu mm (%)	Total Protein Concentration >45 mg/100 ml (%)	Relative IgG Concentration >10.5% (%)	Kappa:Lambda Ratio >1.7 (%)
≤30 (n = 23)	65	65	74	52
31-40 (n = 20)	45	50	85	55
>40 (n = 21)	29	81	62	52

Table 6.—Frequencies of Abnormal MS-CSF Findings in Relation to the Duration of the Disease

Duration (yr)	Mononuclear Leukocytes >5/cu mm (%)	Total Protein Concentration >45 mg/100 ml (%)	Relative IgG Concentration >10.5% (%)	Kappa:Lambda Ratio >1.7 (%)
<1 (n = 8)	63	63	75	63
1-10 (n = 28)	68	61	71	64
>10 (n = 28)	29	71	75	39

terminants may be a valuable laboratory procedure for aiding in establishing a diagnosis of MS.

The increase of kappa: lambda ratio in MS-CSF has been shown to be due probably to a disproportionate increase in the quantity of IgG molecules with light chains of type kappa.[12] In addition, an abnormal electrophoretic distribution of the kappa and lambda light chain antigenic determinants has been demonstrated in CSF-IgG from MS cases in which normal kappa:lambda ratios are found upon inves-

Table 7.—Frequencies of Abnormal MS-CSF Findings in Relation to Length of Interval to Last Exacerbation of the Disease

Interval Between Last Exacerbation and Lumbar Puncture	Mononuclear Cells >5/cu mm (%)	Total Protein Concentration >45 mg/100 ml (%)	Relative IgG Concentration >10.5% (%)	Kappa: Lambda Ratio >1.7 (%)
≦1 mo (n = 29)	62	62	62	55
>1 mo (n = 35)	40	69	83	51

Table 8.—Frequencies of Abnormal MS-CSF Findings in Relation to Disability

Disability Rate	Mononuclear Leukocytes >5/cu mm (%)	Total Protein Concentration >45 mg/100 ml (%)	Relative IgG Concentration >10.5% (%)	Kappa: Lambda Ratio >1.7 (%)
None-slight (n = 43)	60	58	72	58
Moderate-great (n = 21)	29	81	76	43

tigation of unconcentrated CSF samples, indicating that IgG in MS-CSF is oligoclonal.[21] It is possible that the determination of the kappa:lambda ratio of individual γ-globulin fractions obtained by some electrophoretic procedure will be of greater diagnostic value than determination of the kappa:lambda ratio of whole CSF.

Immunoelectrophoresis.—Abnormalities of the IgG precipitation line found on immunoelectrophoresis of MS-CSF have been described under different names. The cathodic extra IgG precipitation line described by Frick[8] in MS and neurosyphilis when using a horse antiserum against human serum is probably identical with the γc-globulin described by Dencker[22] and with the extra precipitation line observed in the cathode in the present investigation. Dencker[22] found this abnormality in 17% of 47 MS cases. This frequency of occurrence is lower than the frequency (31% of 62 MS cases) found in the present investigation.

A doubling of the IgG precipitation line detectable on immunoelectrophoresis of CSF was first described by Laterre et al,[9] who used a horse antiserum against human serum and found this abnormality in 38% of 96 MS cases investigated. Laterre et al[9] also found this abnormality in 28% of 58 samples from patients with infections of the CNS and in 12% of 446 CSF samples from patients with other neurological disorders. This doubling of the IgG precipitation line is probably identical with the γE-globulin described by Dencker[22] when using a rabbit antiserum against human serum and with the "unusual" IgG-globulin described by

MacPherson and Cosgrove[23] when using a horse antiserum against human serum. These investigators found the abnormality in 45% of 47 MS patients[22] and in 36% of 42 MS patients,[23] respectively. The doubling of the IgG precipitation line observed in the present investigation is probably identical with the abnormality described by the above investigators, although it was found to occur somewhat less frequently (26% of 62 MS patients).

The differences in the frequencies of occurrence of these abnormalities demonstrable by immunoelectrophoresis of CSF may be due to differences in the antisera used, as we have observed that various batches of antiserum from the same animal give different results when the same CSF samples were investigated, a finding which considerably reduces the value of the method as a diagnostic tool. The amount of IgG applied as antigen at immunoelectrophoresis seems also to be of importance for the appearance of abnormalities.[10(p88)]

The above-mentioned immunoelectrophoretic abnormalities are rarely seen when serum is investigated. Both occur in neurological disorders other than MS and infectious disorders of the nervous system but with lower frequencies.[9,22] The basic nature of these two CSF abnormalities remains to be elucidated; however, the finding of a doubling of the IgG precipitation line seems to be linked to an abnormal immunoglobulin light chain distribution in CSF.

A finding similar in apppearance to the cathodic extra IgG precipitation line has recently been reported on immunoelec-

132

trophoretic investigation of serum from severely burned patients.[24] The cathodic precipitation line found in these patients seems to be identical with an immunoglobulin component that is comparable with the enzymatically produced F (ab')$_2$ fragment. The occurrence of this immunoglobulin component has been proposed to be the result of an increased in vivo degradation of immunoglobulin due to the larger than normal concentrations of proteolytic enzymes in these patients' sera.

In MS-CSF significantly elevated concentrations of proteolytic enzymes have been found, both in the acute and in the chronic stage of the disease, but especially in the acute stage.[25] The cathodic extra IgG precipitation line found on immunoelectrophoretic investigation of MS-CSF may, therefore, be due to an increased in vivo degradation of IgG. In the present investigation, no correlation was observed between the frequency of occurrence of the cathodic extra IgG precipitation line and the length of interval to last exacerbation of the disease.

Agar Gel Electrophoresis.—Agar gel electrophoresis is clearly the most sensitive of the analytic procedures carried out in the present work for the demonstration of changes in MS-CSF. Among the 64 MS cases studied, it was possible to demonstrate at least two discrete IgG bands in all but four of the cases. In three of these four cases, none of the other investigative procedures was able to detect any CSF abnormalities. In the one remaining case an increased total CSF protein concentration was the only abnormal finding.

The frequency of occurrence (94%) of abnormal CSF agar gel electrophoresis patterns found in MS is close to that previously reported by one of us (H. L.) (100% of 50 cases diagnosed according to the same criteria as in the present investigation)[10] and also to that more recently reported by Laterre et al (86.9% of 84 "definite" MS cases).[11]

It was possible to demonstrate at least two discrete bands in the gamma region in 15 out of 39 CSF samples (39% from patients with infectious disorders of the nervous system, while the corresponding serum electrophoresis patterns were normal in all

Table 9.—CSF Findings in

Case	Age (yr)	Diagnosis	Time Between Debut of Symptoms and Lumbar Puncture (Days)
1	9	Mumps meningitis	10
2	12	Mumps meningitis	1
3	10	Mumps meningitis	17
4	19	Mumps meningitis	50
5	15	Mumps meningitis with hearing loss	4 yr
6	30	Acute aseptic meningitis	1
7	33	Acute aseptic meningitis	14
8	27	Acute aseptic meningitis	2
9	51	Acute aseptic meningitis with bilateral papilledema	90
10	62	Acute aseptic meningitis with paresis of ninth and tenth nerves	14
11	11	Acute aseptic meningitis with paresis of one seventh nerve	7
12	33	Acute aseptic meningitis with paresis of both seventh nerves	12
13	9	Chronic aseptic meningitis	55
14	23	Chronic aseptic meningitis with paresis of sixth nerve	38
15	58	Encephalitis in herpes simplex	19
16	40	Encephalitis in herpes simplex	62
17	48	Meningitis in herpes zoster	45
18	33	Herpes zoster with paresis of third nerve	52

but two of these cases. This finding is in accordance with that of Laterre et al[11] who observed an abnormal agar gel electrophoresis pattern of the CSF γ-globulins in 39.6% of 144 cases with "inflammatory diseases of the CNS."[1]

The nature of the discrete gamma bands occurring in infectious disorders of the nervous system has not been established, in contrast to the discrete CSF gamma bands occurring in MS, which consist of oligoclonal IgG.[10,21] The position of the discrete bands in the infectious disorders is similar to the position of the IgG bands in MS, and it seems most probable that these bands also consist of oligoclonal immunoglobulins. It can, however, not be excluded that the bands sometimes consist of oligoclonal IgA or oligoclonal IgM, at least in those cases in

133

Mononuclear Cells/cu mm	Total Protein Concentration (mg/100 ml)	IgG (%)	IgA (%)	IgM (%)	Kappa: Lambda Ratio	Immuno- electro- phoresis Abnormal*	Agar Gel Electro- phoresis Abnormal†
126	67	7.3	1.3	0.8	0.6	Yes	No
2.150	113	4.7	0.3	<0.25 mg/100 ml	1.2	No	No
30	40	12.2	1.1	<0.25 mg/100 ml	0.3	No	Yes
1	29	6.6	1.8	<0.25 mg/100 ml	0.9	No	No
1	26	8.1	2.6	<0.25 mg/100 ml	1.5	No	No
30	62	...	...	...	...	No	No
165	69	7.0	2.3	<0.25 mg/100 ml	0.4	...	No
86	171	6.3	1.0	0.3	0.9	No	No
116	137	6.9	0.9	<0.25 mg/100 ml	1.2	No	No
61	33	6.4	0.8	<0.25 mg/100 ml	1.1	Yes	No
120	37	10.8	1.2	1.5	0.5	Yes	No
190	36	15.6	1.9	1.1	0.5	No	No
128	117	13.8	1.2	1.7	0.8	Yes	Yes
58	67	5.6	1.3	0.7	1.4	...	No
245	365	29.5	4.9	0.5	1.2	No	Yes
60	168	23.8	1.7	0.2	1.3	No	Yes
29	48	7.7	0.6	<0.25 mg/100 ml	1.3	...	No
23	52	...	...	...	1.1	No	Yes

(Continued on pages 340 and 341.)

which increased relative CSF-IgA or CSF-IgM concentrations are found.

Among the CSF samples from the patients with other neurological disorders, it was possible to demonstrate discrete gamma bands in 3% of the cases. This low frequency of occurrence is consistent with earlier findings.[10,11]

In view of the above findings, it seems reasonable to conclude that, while determination of the CSF kappa:lambda ratio and the relative CSF-IgG concentration may provide supportive information for a diagnosis of MS, agar gel electrophoresis is the most valuable investigative procedure for establishing a diagnosis of MS. Quantitation of CSF-IgA and CSF-IgM and immunoelectrophoresis seem to provide little additional diagnostic information for MS.

It seems probable that the finding of discrete IgG bands on agar gel electrophoresis, increased relative CSF-IgG concentrations, and abnormal kappa:lambda ratios all have the same cause, ie, synthesis of IgG within the CNS. The finding of discrete gamma bands on agar gel electrophoresis and of abnormally high kappa:lambda ratio in addition indicates that the IgG synthesized within the CNS is oligoclonal. The results obtained in the present investigation indicate that the demonstration of oligoclonal CSF-IgG is a more reliable and useful finding in MS than the demonstration of elevated relative CSF-IgG concentration.

It is important to stress that both serum and CSF should always be examined in the agar gel electrophoresis procedure at the same time because electrophoretically homogeneous immunoglobulins (M components) in the serum in myeloma, macroglobulinemia, and other monoclonal gammapathies may migrate into the CSF. In these cases the M components in CSF have the same mobility as they do in serum (Fig 2, D).[26,27] It should be noted, however, that in cases of MS, discrete IgG bands are found only in CSF and not in serum.

Distinct immunoglobulin bands have been demonstrated on agar gel electrophoresis of serum during the course of infections localized outside of the CNS.[28] The low frequency of occurrence of this serum finding may be due to difficulties in discriminating M components from the heavy smear of polyclonal IgG normally found on serum agar gel electrophoresis. This explanation may also be valid for the absence of M components in the agar gel electrophoresis patterns of serum from MS patients and other cases with discrete gamma bands demonstrable on agar gel electrophoresis of CSF.

The appearance of M components in the serum during the course of an infectious disease, eg, malaria,[29] may be attributed to the production of specific antibodies. The function of the electrophoretically homogeneous CSF-IgG in MS and of the electrophoretically homogeneous CSF γ-globulins in infectious disorders of the nervous system and, rarely, in other neurological disorders remains to be elucidated.

The differences found in the present investigation between the CSF findings in MS and in infectious disorders of the nervous system are interesting; however, the similarities between these two groups of disorders in regard to the frequencies of occurrence of the various CSF immunoglobulin abnormalities appear to be of greater significance.

In MS any increase in the CSF concentration of any of the individual immunoglobulins in relation to the total CSF protein concentration is almost always due to IgG, while in infections of the nervous system, the relative CSF concentrations of IgG and/or IgA, sometimes also of IgM, may be found to be increased. This finding and the finding of different frequencies of occurrence of M components, as shown by agar gel electrophoresis, and of abnormal kappa: lambda ratios may indicate that different basic pathogenic mechanisms are involved in

the disease processes.

On the other hand, the fact that similar findings of discrete gamma bands on agar gel electrophoresis are so seldom found in neurological disorders other than MS and infectious disorders of the nervous system lends support to the hypothesis of a common basis to MS and viral CNS infections. The same basic pathogenic and immunological processes may be operating in MS as are believed to be operating in infections of the nervous system.

Relationship Between CSF Findings and Clinical Features in MS.—Increasing total CSF protein concentrations with age have been reported by Cumings.[30] This may at

Table 9.—CSF Findings in

Case	Age (yr)	Diagnosis	Time Between Debut of Symptoms and Lumbar Puncture (Days)
19	59	Herpes zoster with cervical root syndrome	36
20	78	Encephalitis in herpes zoster	6
21	77	Encephalitis in herpes zoster	10
22	77	Herpes zoster	3
23	72	Herpes zoster	9
24	54	Herpes zoster	2 yr
25	61	Herpes zoster	2 yr
26	22	Encephalitis following chicken-pox	9
27	3 mo	Congenital infantile toxoplasmosis	...
28	1 mo	Congenital infantile toxoplasmosis	...
29	9 mo	Acquired infantile toxoplasmosis	...
30	62	Asymptomatic neuro-syphilis	...
31	68	Asymptomatic neuro-syphilis	...
32	32	Asymptomatic neuro-syphilis	...
33	47	Argyll Robertson pupils	...
34	39	Argyll Robertson pupils	...
35	68	Tabes dorsalis	...
36	77	Tabes dorsalis and cerebral hemorrhage	...
37	65	Tabes dorsalis and cerebral hemorrhage	...
38	16	Congenital neurosyphilis	...
39	25	Congenital neurosyphilis	...

Mononuclear Cells/cu mm	Total Protein Concentration (mg/100 ml)	IgG (%)	IgA (%)	IgM (%)	Kappa: Lambda Ratio	Immunoelectrophoresis Abnormal*	Agar Gel Electrophoresis Abnormal†
5	57	7.4	2.1	<0.25 mg/100 ml	0.7	...	No
62	60	13.0	2.7	<0.25 mg/100 ml	1.3	Yes	Yes‡
127	502	12.8	4.3	1.1	1.2	No	No
...	63	7.5	3.8	<0.25 mg/100 ml	0.5	Yes	No
...	69	5.5	2.2	<0.25 mg/100 ml	0.4	No	No
2	44	7.5	1.8	<0.25 mg/100 ml	0.4	No	No
1	66	5.8	<0.2 mg/100 ml	<0.25 mg/100 ml	0.8	...	No
11	44	9.4	0.9	<0.25 mg/100 ml	0.7	No	No
...	1,180	...	...	...	0.6	No	Yes
29	116	...	...	...	...	...	Yes‡
2	34	3.7	<0.2 mg/100 ml	<0.25 mg/100 ml	0.4	No	No
132	119	12.0	1.2	2.3	1.1	No	Yes
1	37	...	...	...	0.5	No	Yes
1	74	10.3	1.0	1.0	1.1	No	Yes
3	55	18.0	0.7	<0.25 mg/100 ml	1.2	No	Yes
6	42	...	...	...	1.0	No	No
...	44	15.9	1.6	<0.25 mg/100 ml	1.3	No	Yes
20	141	7.4	1.2	0.6	0.7	No	No
2	29	5.9	<0.2 mg/100 ml	<0.25 mg/100 ml	0.5	No	No
1	23	14.8	<0.2 mg/100 ml	<0.25 mg/100 ml	1.5	Yes	Yes
1	46	8.0	2.0	<0.25 mg/100 ml	0.7	No	Yes

* "Abnormal" means the presence of an extra IgG precipitation line in the cathode and/or a doubling of the IgG precipitation line.
† "Abnormal" means the presence of at least two discrete bands in the gamma region on agar gel electrophoresis of CSF.
‡ One band in the gamma region of CSF was also visible in the patient's serum.

least in part account for the high frequency of occurrence of elevated total CSF protein concentration found in the present investigation in the group of MS patients with the highest age at the time of lumbar puncture. The finding of a high frequency of occurrence of elevated total CSF protein concentration in the 21 MS patients with moderate or great disability may also partly be due to the over representation of older patients. Only two of the 21 patients were younger than 30 years at the time of lumbar puncture.

Freedman and Merritt found elevated total CSF protein concentrations as often during the first month after an exacerbation of MS symptoms as later.[31] This previous finding is corroborated by the results obtained in the present investigation.

A significantly lower frequency of occurrence of mononuclear pleocytosis was found in the older patients, in the patients with the longest duration of the disease, and in the patient group with the high degree of disability. As previously observed by Freedman and Merritt,[31] there was a difference between the frequency of occurrence of mononuclear pleocytosis in cases investigated within one month after an exacerbation of symptoms and in cases investigated later. This difference was, however, not statistically significant (the difference between the

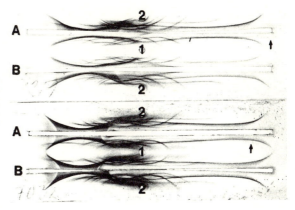

Fig 1.—Immunoelectrophoresis of (1) CSF and (2) serum from patients with MS. Antisera: **A,** antiserum against normal human serum; **B,** antiserum against normal human serum absorbed with light chains. Anode at left.

Fig 2.—Agar gel electrophoresis of (1) CSF and (2) serum from **A,** healthy control; **B** and **C,** two patients with MS; **D,** a patient with benign, essential monoclonal gammapathy. **Arrows** pointing downward denote IgG; **arrows** pointing upward denote beta-trace protein to left of IgG and gamma-trace protein to right of IgG. Anode at left.

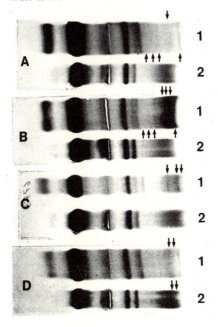

percentages was 1.8 times the standard error giving $0.05 < P < 0.1$), but the patient groups were small.

Yahr et al[3] found no correlation between the duration of the disease and the frequency of occurrence of increased relative CSF-IgG concentration. These previous findings are supported by the results obtained in the present investigation.

Yahr et al[3] did not find any difference in the frequency of occurrence of increased relative CSF-IgG concentration when comparing cases investigated within one month after an exacerbation of symptoms and cases investigated later.[3] In the present investigation a difference was found between the percentages of increased relative CSF-IgG concentration in these two groups of patients. However, this difference was not statistically significant (the difference was 1.9 times the standard error giving $0.05 < P < 0.1$). This finding of lowered relative CSF-IgG concentrations in relation to an exacerbation of the disease may be due to increased "consumption" of IgG or may be due to a temporary blockade in synthesis of IgG. Quantitation of IgG in consecutive CSF samples from individual MS patients during exacerbations and during the chronic phase of the disease may throw further light on the question of alterations of the relative CSF-IgG concentration during the disease process.

The frequency of occurrence of abnormally high CSF kappa:lambda ratio seems to vary only along one of the four clinical

137

factors investigated as it was found to be significantly higher in patients investigated within ten years after onset when compared with those with a longer duration of the disease.

Conclusions

Using an immunodiffusion technique suitable for the quantitation of individual proteins in unconcentrated CSF, relative CSF IgG concentrations (expressed in percent of the total CSF protein concentration) were found to be increased in 73% of the 64 MS-CSF samples investigated. The relative CSF IgA concentrations were found to be increased in only 9% of the samples, and the relative CSF IgM concentrations were not elevated in any of the cases studied. The serum IgG, IgA, and IgM concentrations were nearly all within normal limits. Oligoclonal CSF-IgG was found among the MS-CSF samples in the form of discrete bands on agar gel electrophoresis in 94% of the cases and in the form of abnormalities in the ratio of light chains of type kappa to light chains of type lambda in 53% of the cases, while the corresponding serum findings were normal in all cases investigated.

In the analysis of CSF samples from 39 patients with infectious disorders of the nervous system, increased relative IgG, IgA, and IgM concentrations were found in 36%, 27%, and 9% of the cases, respectively, while the corresponding serum findings were nearly all within normal limits. Discrete bands in the gamma region on agar gel electrophoresis were found in 39% of these cases, while the kappa:lambda ratios and corresponding serum findings were normal in all.

Among 81 CSF samples from patients with other neurological disorders, increased relative IgG, IgA, and IgM concentrations were found in 16%, 14%, and 6%, respectively. Discrete bands in the gamma region on agar gel electrophoresis and abnormal kappa:lambda ratios were found in only 3% of these cases.

Agar gel electrophoresis, which has been shown to be the most sensitive electrophoresis technique presently available for the demonstration of discrete IgG bands in CSF, is shown in the present investigation also to be the most valuable CSF investigative procedure for establishing a diagnosis of MS. Quantitation of individual immunoglobulins and immunoelectrophoresis provide little diagnostic information beyond that obtained by agar gel electrophoresis, while the determination of the kappa:lambda ratio may differentiate between MS and viral infections of the central nervous system.

The CSF abnormalities in MS are correlated to different clinical factors.

This investigation was supported by grants from the Swedish Multiple Sclerosis Society.

References

1. Kabat EA, Glusman M, Knaub V: Quantitative estimation of the albumin and gammaglobulin in normal and pathologic cerebrospinal fluid by immunochemical methods. *Amer J Med* 4:653-662, 1948.

2. Kabat EA, Freedman DA, Murray JP, et al: A study of the crystalline albumin, gamma globulin and total protein in the cerebrospinal fluid of one hundred cases of multiple sclerosis and in other diseases. *Amer J Med Sci* 219:55-64, 1950.

3. Yahr MD, Goldensohn SS, Kabat EA: Further studies on the gamma globulin content of cerebrospinal fluid in multiple sclerosis and other neurological diseases. *Ann NY Acad Sci* 58:613-624, 1954.

4. Hartley TF, Merrill DA, Claman HN: Quantitation of immunoglobulins in cerebrospinal fluid. *Arch Neurol* 15:472-479, 1966.

5. Bauer HJ, Gottesleben A: Quantitative immunochemical studies of cerebrospinal fluid proteins in relation to clinical activity of multiple sclerosis, in Pathogenesis and etiology of demyelinating diseases. *Int Arch Allerg* 36:643-648, 1969.

6. Kabat EA, Moore DH, Landow H: An electrophoretic study of the protein components in cerebrospinal fluid and their relationship to the serum proteins. *J Clin Invest* 21:571-577, 1942.

7. Uyeda CT, Gerstl B, Eng LF, et al: Serum immunoglobulins in multiple sclerosis patients. *Proc Soc Exp Biol Med* 131:1138-1141, 1969.

8. Frick E: Immunophoretische Untersuchungen am Liquor cerebrospinalis. *Klin Wschr* 37:645-651, 1959.

9. Laterre EC, Heremans JF, Demanet G: La pathologie des protéines du liquide céphalo-rachidien. *Rev Neurol* 107:500-521, 1962.

10. Link H: Immunoglobulin G and low molecular weight proteins in human cerebrospinal fluid: Chemical and immunological characterisation with special reference to multiple sclerosis. *Acta Neurol Scand* 43(suppl 28):1-136, 1967.

11. Laterre EC, Callewaert A, Heremans JF, et al: Electrophoretic morphology of gamma globulins in cerebrospinal fluid of multiple sclerosis and other diseases of the nervous system. *Neurology* **20**:982-990, 1970.

12. Link H, Zettervall O: Multiple Sclerosis: Disturbed kappa:lambda light chain ratio of immunoglobulin G in cerebrospinal fluid. *Clin Exp Immun* **6**:435-438, 1970.

13. Müller R: Studies on multiple sclerosis. *Acta Med Scand* **133**(suppl 222):1-214, 1949.

14. Norberg R: The immunoglobulin content of normal serum. *Acta Med Scand* **181**:485-496, 1967.

15. Lous P, Plum CM, Schou M: Colorimetric determination of total protein and globulin in cerebrospinal fluid. *Nord Med* **55**:693-695, 1956.

16. Schneck SA, Claman HN: CSF immunoglobulins in multiple sclerosis and other neurologic diseases: Measurement by electroimmunodiffusion. *Arch Neurol* **20**:132-139, 1969.

17. Riddoch D, Thompson RA: Immunoglobulin levels in the cerebrospinal fluid. *Brit Med J* **1**:396-399, 1970.

18. Link H, Zettervall O: Increased cerebrospinal fluid (CSF) total protein, a sign of blood CSF-barrier damage: Report, in Paoletti R (ed): *Second International Meeting of the International Society for Neurochemistry.* Milan, Italy, Tamburini Editore, 1969, pp 269-270.

19. Cohen S, Bannister R: Immunoglobulin synthesis within the central nervous system in multiple sclerosis. *Lancet* **1**:366-367, 1967.

20. Frick E, Scheid-Seydel L: Untersuchungen mit J¹³¹-markiertem γ-Globulin zur Frage der Abstammung der Liquoreiweisskörper. *Klin Wschr* **36**:857-863, 1958.

21. Zettervall O, Link H: Electrophoretic distribution of kappa and lambda immunoglobulin light chain determinants in serum and CSF in multiple sclerosis. *Clin Exp Immun* **7**:365-372, 1970.

22. Dencker J: Immunoelectrophoretic investigation of cerebrospinal fluid γ-globulins in multiple sclerosis. *Acta Neurol Scand* **40**(suppl 10):57-64, 1964.

23. MacPherson CFC, Cosgrove JBR: An unusual IgG globulin: Frequency of occurrence in cerebrospinal fluid in multiple sclerosis. *Arch Neurol* **19**:503-509, 1968.

24. Goldberg CB, Whitestone F: F(ab¹)₂-like fragments from severely burned patients provide a new serum immunoglobulin component. *Nature* **228**:160-162, 1970.

25. Rinne UK, Riekkinen P: Esterase, peptidase and proteinase activities of human cerebrospinal fluid in multiple sclerosis. *Acta Neurol Scand* **44**:156-167, 1968.

26. Wallenius G: Electrophoretic patterns of cerebrospinal fluid and serum compared in normal and pathological conditions. *Acta Soc Med Upsal* **57**:138-146, 1952.

27. Weiss AH, Smith E, Cristoff N, et al: Cerebrospinal fluid paraproteins in multiple myeloma. *J Lab Clin Med* **66**:280-293, 1965.

28. Michaux J-L, Heremans JF: Thirty cases of monoclonal immunoglobulin disorders other than myeloma or macroglobulinemia. *Amer J Med* **46**:562-579, 1969.

29. Hällén J: Discrete gammaglobulin (M-) components in serum. *Acta Med Scand* **179**(suppl 462):1-427, 1966.

30. Cumings JN: The cerebrospinal fluid in diagnosis. *Brit Med J* **1**:449-451, 1954.

31. Freedman DA, Merritt HH: The cerebrospinal fluid in multiple sclerosis. *Res Publ Assoc Res Nerv Ment Dis* **28**:428-439, 1950.

Antibody to Encephalitogenic Basic Protein in Multiple Sclerosis and other Neurological Diseases as Measured by Immune Adherence

E. A. Caspary and M. E. Chambers

The possibility that autoimmune phenomena may be involved in the pathogenesis of certain diseases of the human central nervous system [reviewed by Paterson, 1965, 1966] has led to many attempts to demonstrate antibody (factors) in the serum of patients capable of combining specifically with constituents of the nervous system. This search for serum factors has yielded a conflicting series of results, related both to method and the precise nature of the antigen employed [Lisak et al., 1968; Caspary, 1968] and no reaction specific only to demyelinating disorders, as typified by multiple sclerosis (MS), has yet been demonstrated.

The present study reports a further attempt to detect specific serum factors to encephalitogenic basic protein (EF) in patients with MS, neurological disease other than multiple sclerosis and in normal healthy individuals by the method of immune adherence [Turk, 1964].

Materials and Methods

Sera from 20 cases of acute MS, 8 of chronic MS and 32 patients suffering from other neurological diseases were studied. The normal control group (24) consisted of laboratory staff and blood donors, 16 males and 8 females with a mean age of 33. The group of acute MS patients had equal numbers of males and females with a mean age of 37 and the chronic cases had 3 males and 5 females of average age 43. Other neurological diseases were split into 2 groups; one of general paralysis of the insane 7 females and 9 males, mean age 56, and a miscellaneous group, 10 males and 6 females, mean age 50 (polyneuropathy 5, motor neurone disease 4, cerebral tumour 2, transverse myelitis 1, craniopharyngioma 1, Jacob-Creutzfeld 1, presenile dementia 1, cerebellar degeneration 1).

Tests for antibody to EF were performed by the immune adherence technique as described by TURK [1964]. To 0.2 ml vol of doubling dilutions of serum in veronal-saline with added Ca and Mg [KABAT and MAYER, 1961] in 80×12 mm tubes were added 0.5 ml antigen (EF 5 μg/ml) and 0.2 ml of preserved guinea-pig complement. Optimal antigen and complement concentrations were determined by a chequer-board titration as described in the original method, sera were heated at 56° C for 30 min to inactivate complement before testing. The mixture was incubated at 37° C followed by the addition of 0.1 ml of 1.5 % (v/v) washed human red cells (group 0) and a further incubation for 60 min at 37° C. At the end of the second incubation the haemagglutination patterns in the tubes were read, doubtful patterns of the $\pm$ type were taken as negative.

To confirm the specificity of the reaction, sera were absorbed with either brain powder or kidney powder at room temperature for 30 min, centrifuged at 1,000 g for 8 min and the clear supernatant tested as above. The soluble nature of EF did not permit absorption with specific antigen alone, as this leaves excess antigen free in the supernate.

Results

The results of immune adherence titrations are shown in table I. It will be seen that titres in acute MS are significantly greater than those in normal controls (P 0.01) and that other neurological disease (P 0.001) and general paralysis of the insane (GPI) (P 0.001) also showed a significant increase. The small number of chronic MS patients studied had increased titres but failed to reach an acceptable level of statistical significance (P 0.1). There were no significant differences between acute and chronic MS, or between MS and other neurological disease, though the mean titre in GPI was significantly greater than in MS (0.02, P 0.01).

Absorbtion with brain markedly reduced the titres (table II) but only minimal change was obtained with a non-specific tissue powder (kidney).

Discussion

Immune adherence titres against EF were increased both in MS and in other degenerative neurological disease, especially in GPI.

These findings are in full agreement with a number of other studies which failed to demonstrate disease specific 'antibody' to either brain or brain fractions [reviewed LISAK et al., 1968]. These authors also suggest that there is no antibody to EF in any human neurological disorder with

141

Table I. Antibodies to EF tested by immune adherence

	Normal	Acute MS	Chronic MS	GPI	Other neurological diseases
No. of cases	24	20	8	16	16
Mean Titre (tubes of doubling dilution)	3.20	4.95	4.37	6.68	5.50
± Standard error	0.30	0.54	0.74[1]	0.27	0.53
Statistical comparison		vs normal P 0.01	vs normal not significant	vs normal P 0.001	vs normal P 0.001
			vs acute MS not significant	vs acute MS 0.02, P 0.01	vs acute MS not significant
					vs GPI not significant

[1] Cochran's correction for unequal variance applied.

Table II. Effect of absorbtion with brain and kidney powder with brain and kidney powder on immune adherence titres

	Sera		
	MS 1	MS 2	MS 3
Unabsorbed	6	7	4
Brain powder	1	2	0
Kidney powder	5	5	3

Titres are expressed as tubes of doubling dilution.

the very sensitive method of radio-immunoelectrophoresis using ^{125}I labelled antigen and similar attempts using the FARR technique also proved negative. It is unlikely that these findings could be attributed to unstable radio-labelled material [CASPARY and FIELD, 1968]. However, failure to demonstrate antibody by one method does not entirely invalidate positive results obtained with others.

The question then arises whether the reacting factor measured is antibody globulin or some other component of serum capable of combining specifically with antigens. In many of the studies carried out in MS [FIELD, 1965] similar responses were obtained with sera from patients with other nervous diseases, rheumatoid arthritis or Hashimoto's disease and low titres of 'antibody' were shown even in the serum of normal individuals; this situation has its parallel in Hashimoto's thyroiditis where low titre antibody can be shown in nearly half the population and only very high values are considered pathological. The nature and function of 'antibody' demonstrated by several different methods can only ultimately be demonstrated by assessment of its biological function, and the protective action of complement fixing antibody to brain in allergic encephalomyelitis [PATERSON and HARWIN, 1963] suggests that, at least in experimental animals, these antibodies play some definite part in the disease process. The reaction with EF can be shown to be specific and it is suggested that this results from antibody (or serum factor) produced following the release of material from an immunologically privileged site, caused by disease in the 'target organ'.

References

CASPARY, E. A.: Demyelinating diseases and allergic encephalomyelitis. A comparative review with special reference to multiple sclerosis; in CUMINGS and KREMER. Biochemical aspects of neurological disorders, 3rd series, p. 44 (Blackwell, Oxford 1968).

CASPARY, E. A. and FIELD, E. J.: Stability of radioiodinated encephalitogenic factor *in vivo*. Clin. exp. Immunol. *3:* 747 (1968).

FIELD, E. J.: Some observations on the clinical immunology of multiple sclerosis; in slow, latent and temperate virus infections; NINDB Monograph No. 2, p. 187 (1965).

KABAT, E. A. and MAYER, M. M.: in experimental immunochemistry, p. 149 (Thomas, Springfield 1961).

LISAK, R. P.; HEINZE, R. G.; FALK, G. A. and KIES, M. W.: Search for antiencephalitogen antibody in human demyelinative disease. Neurology, Minneap. *18:* 122 (1968).

PATERSON, P. Y.: in SAMTER Immunological diseases, p. 788 (Little, Brown, Boston 1965).

PATERSON, P. Y. and HARWIN, S. M.: Suppression of allergic encephalomyelitis by means of antibrain serum. J. exp Med. *117:* 755 (1963).

PATERSON, P. Y.: Experimental allergic encephalomyelitis and autoimmune disease. Adv. Immunol. *5:* 131 (1966).

TURK, J. L.: The detection of antibodies by immune adherence; in ACKROYD Immunological methods, p. 405 (Blackwell, Oxford 1964).

Serum and cerebrospinal fluid immunoglobulins in multiple sclerosis

Oldrich J. Kolar, M.D., Alexander T. Ross, M.D.,

and Jean T. Herman, M.D.

Since the communication of Kabat et al.,[1] an elevation of the electrophoretically determined fraction of the cerebrospinal fluid (CSF) gamma globulins has been recognized as a concomitant of multiple sclerosis (MS). It was further demonstrated[2] that there is a positive correlation between the concentration of the CSF immunoglobulin-G (IgG) and the increased amount of this immunoglobulin in the plaques of MS patients. By means of immunofluorescent techniques, Simpson et al.[3] showed that the highest concentration of IgG appeared in the margin of active plaques. However, Tourtellotte and Parker[2] also reported about 2.7 times higher concentration of IgG in the normal appearing white matter of the brains from MS patients compared with controls. Increased IgG concentration was further demonstrated in brain extracts in subacute sclerosing panencephalitis,[4] in Huntington's chorea, and in multiple myeloma.[5] Thus, elevated IgG concentration in brain tissue extracts, as in the CSF,[6–8] is not pathognomonic of MS.

In agreement with the generally accepted opinion that the immunoglobulins are formed by the lymphoid cell system,[9] Cohen and Bannister[10] and Sandberg-Wollheim et al.[11] indicate that the local production of IgG and immunoglobulin-A (IgA) in the CNS tissue structures is carried in MS by immunologically competent mononuclear cells. In these experimental studies, the lymphoid cells were recovered from the CSF and cultured in vitro. In addition, it was shown by Cohen and Bannister[10] that these cells have produced increased amounts of the kappa light polypeptide chains. Increased kappa to lambda light chain ratio was subsequently observed by Zetterval and Link[12] in CSF specimens from 6 of the 11 MS patients with M components in the CSF gamma globulin region.

On the other hand, there is as yet no evidence that in MS patients the CSF IgG differs in Gm and Inv typing from the serum IgG.[13] Nor has it so far been established which proportion of the immunocompetent cells producing immunoglobulins in the CNS of MS patients, directly or as daughter generations, originate from the extraneural lymphoreticular structures. There are, however, experimental indications that in patients with clinically active MS, mononuclear blood cells may attack glia cells in tissue cultures.[14]

Important observations in chronic inflammatory and demyelinating CNS afflictions, including MS, were brought out by CSF and serum agar gel and cellulose polyacetate electrophoresis. Lowenthal et al.[15] and Laterre,[16] using agar gel electrophoresis, demonstrated one to four protein bands in the CSF gamma globulin field of MS patients. In MS, as in subacute sclerosing panencephalitis (SSPE), two of these M-type gamma globulin components were encountered most commonly in

CSF electropherograms.[17] However, in SSPE the M components in the CSF gamma globulin region usually appeared in a more cathodal position, were more distinct, and were demonstrated in higher numbers. In addition, Lowenthal et al.[18] demonstrated these M components in the gamma globulin region of the serum electropherograms of patients with SSPE. Up to six M components exhibiting very similar electrophoretic mobility in the serum and CSF electropherograms can be demonstrated in SSPE patients by means of cellulose polyacetate electrophoresis.[19]

In 1964 Dencker reported immunoelectrophoretic studies in 47 patients with MS.[20] By means of modified Scheidegger's micromethod[21] an elongation of the anodal segment and the appearance of the gamma-E and the gamma-C component of the IgG precipitate in the CSF immunoelectropherograms of MS patients were demonstrated. Using anti-CSF antiserum, Dencker[20] showed an anodal extension of both the 7S gamma-1 and the 7S gamma-2 precipitates in the CSF specimens from MS patients. In addition to the abnormalities in the CSF IgG precipitation arc, he also reported an extension and an increased density of the IgA precipitate and the presence of the precipitation arc of immunoglobulin-M (IgM) in the CSF immunoelectropherograms of the MS cases studied. Using the immunodiffusion method, Bauer et al.[22] detected CSF IgM in over 30% of their 70 cases of MS. This is in agreement with the observation that immunodiffusion methods appear to be more reliable in the detection of immunoglobulins.[23] On the other hand, immunoelectrophoresis remains the most sensitive method for demonstration of qualitative abnormalities of immunoglobulins.[24] It should be pointed out, however, that the qualitative changes in CSF immunoglobulins demonstrated in MS patients were also detected in a wide variety of subacute or chronic inflammatory and demyelinating CNS afflictions.

While qualitative and quantitative abnormalities in the CSF immunoglobulins in MS patients have been intensively studied, changes in the serum immunoglobulins have attracted less attention. Using paper electrophoresis, Szabo[25] found an increase of serum gamma globulins primarily in patients suffering from the chronic form of MS, while the deviations in the alpha$_1$- glyco- and lipoproteins were more marked in acute exacerbations of the disease. Agar gel electrophoresis did not reveal M components in the serum gamma globulin field of the MS patients.[17] However, using serum immunoelectrophoresis, Clausen[26] reported findings reflecting a "mobilization of the immune apparatus" in MS patients as manifested by hyperimmunoglobulinemia. Qualitative abnormalities in the serum IgG precipitate were later immunoelectrophoretically demonstrated by Kolar[27] in cases of SSPE. A split in the cathodal segment of the serum IgG precipitation arc or the appearance of the so called gamma-C determinant was also reported by Cutler et al.[28] A split in the cathodal segment or the gamma-C determinant or both, together with other abnormalities in serum IgG precipitate, were further immunoelectrophoretically demonstrated in MS and in a variety of subacute inflammatory or demyelinating CNS afflictions.[29]

More pronounced qualitative abnormalities in the CSF and serum IgG precipitates in SSPE and MS patients were revealed when anti-Fc fragments and anti-Fab fragments antisera were used in immunoelectrophoretic examinations.[30,31] It was shown that the more cathodally situated component in the split cathodal segment of the serum or CSF or both IgG precipitate usually exhibited a corresponding position with the cathodal end of the precipitate demonstrated in the same specimens with the antiserum against the Fab fragments of IgG. The immunochemical studies done by Bergmann et al.[32] also suggested that the gamma-C determinant of IgG is made up of several components of small molecular size which bear antigenic relationship to the Fab fragments of IgG. Using the electroimmunodiffusion (EID) method,[33] a higher concentration of the serum and CSF Fab fragments of IgG was found in MS and different subacute inflammatory or demyelinating CNS diseases compared with CNS afflictions without significant subacute or chronic inflammatory and demyelinating manifestations.[31,34]

It is the purpose of this paper to compare abnormal electrophoretic and immunoelectrophoretic findings in serum and CSF of 64 patients with MS. In addition, CSF cytomorphol-

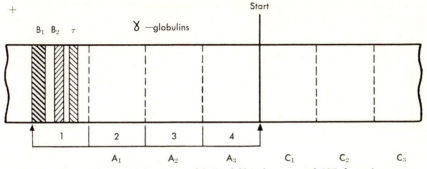

Fig. 1. Schematic division of the gamma globulins field in the serum and CSF electropherograms

ogy and the concentration of serum and CSF immunoglobulins were also examined.

MATERIALS AND METHODS

From 102 patients diagnosed as having MS, 64 were selected as definite MS cases. The table contains information about the sex and age distribution, the time elapsed from the appearance of the first clinical symptomatology, and the course of the disease at the time the spinal tap was performed.

The CSFs were obtained by lumbar puncture and stored without preservatives together with the serum at 4° C. Examinations of CSF and serum specimens were completed within four to twelve days. The total protein concentration was determined photometrically or by the ultraviolet spectrophotometric method or both.[35] The CSF was concentrated by ultrafiltration at 4° C. The serum and concentrated CSF specimens were electrophoretically examined by means of cellulose polyacetate electrophoresis in cooled chambers using tris-barbital-sodium buffer pH 8.8, 0.05 μ. Current of 2.4 to 2.6 milliamperes per strip was applied for one hundred and twenty minutes. The strips were then stained with Ponceau S red, and the protein bands were eluted in 0.1 sodium hydroxide. The optical density of the sample was determined in a Cary 15 spectrophotometer or the strips were evaluated densimetrically or both. The position of M components are shown on the schematic drawing of Figure 1. The application line, representing the starting point of the serum and CSF electropherograms, indicates the border between the anodal A_3 and the first cathodal C_1 segment of the gamma globulin region.

Modified Scheidegger's micromethod[21] (solution of 1.5% agar in sodium barbital buffer of pH 8.8, 0.05 μ) was applied for immunoelectrophoretic examinations. Antihuman rabbit antiserum and monovalent antiserums (anti-hemopexin, IgG, IgM, IgA, and immunoglobulin-D (IgD) antiserums, antiserum against Fab fragments of the IgG and against the kappa and lambda polypeptide chains were used. Two to six immunoelectrophoretic examinations of the serum and the CSF specimens were performed in each of the MS patients studied.

Serum IgG, IgA, IgM, and IgD levels were examined by radial immunodiffusion method. Normal variations in serum IgG, IgA, and IgM concentration were determined by examination of 58 healthy blood donors and are recorded in the table ($\bar{x} \pm 2_s \pm 10\%$ for technical errors). The concentration of CSF IgG, IgA, and IgM was determined by means of EID.[36] From our experience in over 2,200 examinations of the IgG, IgA, and IgM levels in tissue extracts and CSF specimens, the range of technical errors using the EID method represents $\pm$ 5 to 22%.

CSF cytomorphology was studied using a sedimentation apparatus.[37]

RESULTS

Abnormal electrophoretic, immunoelectrophoretic, and cytological findings, together with concentration of the serum and CSF immunoglobulins beyond the range of normal variations. are summarized on the table. As

147

Total number of males (M)		33	51.6%
Total number of females (F)		31	48.4%

Representation of patients by age groups —

(M)	10-19 years	1	1.5%
(F)	10-19 years	1	1.5%
(M)	20-29 years	14	21.8%
(F)	20-29 years	13	20.3%
(M)	30-39 years	10	15.6%
(F)	30-39 years	10	15.6%
(M)	40-49 years	6	9.3%
(F)	40-49 years	6	9.3%
(M)	50-59 years	0	
(F)	50-59 years	0	
(M)	60-up years	2	3.1%
(F)	60-up years	1	1.5%

Time elapsed from the appearance
of the first clinical symptomatology —

Less than 1 year	6	9.3%
1-2 years	14	21.8%
3-4 years	13	20.3%
5-6 years	8	12.5%
7-8 years	4	6.2%
9-10 and over 10 years	15	23.4%
No reliable clinical history	4	6.2%

Course of the disease —

Course with remissions, progressive phase	34	53.1%
Course with remissions, stabilized phase	7	10.9%
Course with remissions, regressive phase	1	1.5%
Acute phase (first episode)	5	7.8%
Chronic-progressive course	14	21.8%
No reliable clinical history	3	4.6%

Abnormal urine findings	9.7%
White blood cells over 10,000 per cubic millimeter	28.9%

SERUM

(1) Serum total proteins over 8%	4.7%

A. Electrophoretic abnormalities

(2) Albumin concentration over 65% of total proteins	10.9%
Albumin concentration below 45% of total proteins	12.5%
(3) Concentration of alpha-1 globulins over 8% of total proteins	7.8%
2 bands in the region of alpha-1 globulins	4.6%
3 bands in the region of alpha-1 globulins	0 %
(4) Concentration of alpha-2 globulins over 14% of total proteins	14.0%
3 bands in the region of alpha-2 globulins	7.8%
4 bands and more in the region of alpha-2 globulins	3.1%
Alpha-2 globulins over 14% and/or 3 and more bands in the alpha-2 globulins region	17.0%
(5) Concentration of beta globulins over 15% of total proteins	9.3%
3 bands in the region of beta globulins	12.5%
4 bands and more in the region of beta globulins	1.5%
Beta globulins over 15% and/or 3 and more bands in the beta globulin region	15.6%
(6) Concentration of gamma globulins over 20% of total proteins	14.0%

(7) 1 M component in the gamma globulins region	A1	1.5%
	A2	4.6%
	A3	4.6%
	C1	1.5%
	C2	0 %
2 M components in the gamma globulins region	A1, A2	1.5%
	A2, A3	12.5%
	A3, C1	0 %
	C1, C2	1.5%
3 M components in the gamma globulins region	A1, A2, A3	1.5%

1-3 M components in the gamma globulins region	28.1%
Concentration of gamma globulins over 20% of total proteins and/or presence of M components in the gamma globulin region	35.9%

M components showing the corresponding electrophoretic mobility in serum and CSF independent from the additional M components in the CSF electropherogram	A1	1.5%
	A2	3.1%
	A3	3.1%
	C1	0 %
	C2	0 %
	A1, A2	0 %
	A2, A3	10.9%
	A3, C1	0 %
	C1, C2	1.5%

B. Immunoelectrophoretic abnormalities

(8)	IgG	40.6%
	"Shadow" formation	37.5%
	Longitudinal split (gamma-E fraction)	1.5%
	Split in the cathodal segment	9.5%
(9)	Fab fragments of IgG	35.9%
	"Shadow" formation	14.2%
	Longitudinal split	3.1%
	Split in the cathodal segment	6.3%
	Increased density of the cathodal segment of the precipitate	11.1%
	Increased density of the anodal segment of the precipitate	3.1%
(10)	IgA	23.4%
	"Shadow" formation	10.9%
	"Fuzziness" in the cathodal segment	10.9%
(11)	IgM	6.2%
	"Shadow" formation	3.1%
	Increased density of the cathodal segment	1.5%
	"Fuzziness" in the cathodal segment	1.5%
	"Shadow" formation in the IgG precipitate showing the same immunoelectrophoretic mobility as the "shadow" formation in CSF IgG precipitation arc	26.5%
	Split in the cathodal segment of the precipitate of the Fab fragments of IgG with the corresponding immunoelectrophoretic findings in the CSF Fab precipitate	3.1%
	Longitudinal split (1 to 3 gamma-E fractions) in the precipitate of Fab fragments showing identical electrophoretic mobility and configuration of the precipitation arc in serum and CSF	3.1%

C. Concentration of immunoglobulins

Normal variations (± 10% for technical errors)
IgG   1359 ± 342 mg./100 ml.
IgA   196 ± 157 mg./100 ml.
IgM   90 ± 56 mg./100 ml.

(12)	IgG: over 1,871 mg./100 ml.	12.3%
	Below 600 mg./100 ml.	0 %
(13)	IgA: over 388 mg./100 ml.	13.8%
	Below 35 mg./100 ml.	1.5%
(14)	IgM: over 161 mg./100 ml.	7.8%
	Below 34 mg./100 ml.	3.1%

(15)	IgD: 29 mg./100 ml. and over	6.4%
	Patients with increased concentration of:	
	IgG and IgA	7.8%
	IgG and IgM	3.1%
	IgA and IgM	3.1%
	IgG, IgA, and IgM	1.5%
	IgG, IgA, and IgD	1.5%
	Patients with abnormal concentration in IgG, IgA, and/or IgM	33.8%

CEREBROSPINAL FLUID

(16)	Cell count of 3 or more cells in 1 cu. mm.	39.1%
	Cell count of 5 or more cells in 1 cu. mm.	26.6%
	Cell count of 10 or more cells in 1 cu. mm.	11.1%
(17)	Plsama cells in CSF cytograms	54.0%
(18)	Reticulomonocytes over 35%	22.9%
	Reticulomonocytes over 35% together with plasma cells	6.4%
(19)	Total protein concentration over 50 mg./100 ml.	35.4%
(20)	Parenchymal type of the colloidal gold reaction	66.6%

A. Electrophoresis

(21)	Albumin concentration over 65% of total proteins	7.8%
	Albumin concentration below 45% of total proteins	18.7%
(22)	Concentration of alpha-1 globulins over 7% of total proteins	10.9%
	2 bands in the region of alpha-1 globulins	9.3%
(23)	Concentration of alpha-2 globulins over 8% of total proteins	26.5%
	3 bands in the region of alpha-2 globulins	7.8%
	4 bands in the region of alpha-2 globulins	6.2%
	Concentration of alpha-2 globulins over 8% of total proteins and/or 3 and more bands in the alpha-2 globulins region	28.1%
(24)	Concentration of beta globulins over 16% of total proteins	7.8%
	3 bands in the region of beta globulins	13.1%
	Concentration of the Tau fraction mounting over 50% of the level of the beta-1 fraction	42.1%

(25) Gamma/beta globulin ratio over 1   76.6%

(26) Concentration of gamma globulins:

Over 12% of total proteins	79.3%
Over 14% of total proteins	58.7%
Over 16% of total proteins	53.1%
Over 18% of total proteins	39.6%
Over 20% of total proteins	26.9%
Over 22% of total proteins	25.3%
Over 26% of total proteins	14.2%
Over 30% of total proteins	9.5%

(27) M components in the gamma globulin region   68.8%

1 M components	A1	0 %
	A2	11.1%
	A3	6.3%
	C1	0 %
	C2	0 %
2 M components	A1, A2	3.1%
	A2, A3	15.8%
	A3, C1	6.3%
	C1, C2	0 %
3 M components	A1, A2, A3	4.7%
	A2, A3, C1	9.5%
	A3, C1, C2	3.1%
4 M components	A1, A2, A3, C1	1.5%
5 M components	A1, A2, A3, C1, C2	1.5%

Elevated concentration of gamma globulins over 12% of total protein amount and/or presence of M components in the gamma globulin region   88.8%

Presence of M components in CSF specimens with the gamma globulin concentration below 12% of the total protein amount   11.1%

B. Immunoelectrophoretic abnormalities

(28) Albumin precipitate   15.8%

Cathodal elongation	7.9%
Deconfiguration of the cathodal segment	3.1%
Split in the cathodal segment	4.7%

(29) IgG   80.9%

"Shadow" formation	71.4%
Cathodal elongation	55.5%
Anodal elongation	20.6%
Longitudinal split (gamma-E fraction)	22.2%
Split in the cathodal segment (gamma-C fraction)	14.2%

(30) Fab fragments of IgG   47.6%

"Shadow" formation	9.5%
Longitudinal split	6.3%
Split in the cathodal segment	22.2%
Cathodal elongation	11.1%
Anodal elongation	4.7%

(31) IgA   17.4%

"Shadow" formation	4.7%
Longitudinal split	1.5%
Cathodal elongation	12.6%

(32) IgM—presence of the precipitate   10.6%

(33) Hemopexin—cathodal displacement of the precipitation arc   18.1%

(34) Abnormal staining patterns in the gamma globulin region   39.6%

Abnormal staining patterns in a corresponding position in both the CSF and the serum immunoelectropherograms   15.6%

C. Concentration of immunoglobulins

(35) IgG—over 4 mg./100 ml.   77.7%

(36) IgA—over 0.6 mg./100 ml.   35.9%

(37) IgM—detected   26.9%

Increased concentration of the IgG over 4 mg./100 ml. and/or immunoelectrophoretic abnormalities in the IgG precipitate   95.1%

Increased concentration of the IgG over 4 mg./100 ml. and/or elevation of the gamma globulins over 12% of the total protein amount   93.7%

Increased concentration of the IgG over 4 mg./100 ml. and/or presence of M components in the gamma globulin region   92.0%

Increased concentration of the IgG over 4 mg./100 ml. in absence of M components in the gamma globulin region   18.7%

Increased concentration of the IgG over 4 mg./100 ml. in CSF specimens with the gamma globulin level below 12% of the total protein   12.6%

Presence of M components in the gamma globulin region in CSF specimens with the concentration of the IgG below 4 mg./100 ml.   7.9%

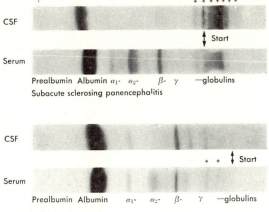

Cellulose polyacetate electrophoresis

+   * * * * * * *

CSF

                                     ↕ Start

Serum

Prealbumin Albumin α₁- α₂- β- γ —globulins
Subacute sclerosing panencephalitis

CSF

                                     * * ↕ Start

Serum

Prealbumin Albumin   α₁- α₂- β- γ —globulins

Multiple sclerosis

Fig. 2. Cerebrospinal fluid (CSF) and serum electropherograms in a 5-year-old girl with subacute sclerosing panencephalitis and in a 27-year-old man with multiple sclerosis. The electrophoretic mobility of M components is indicated by asterisks (*).

indicated by numbers, there were thirty-seven aspects analyzed, each usually with a few subgroups.

Figure 2 represents relatively typical position of M components in the gamma globulin regions of the CSF and serum electropherograms in SSPE and MS. The electrophoretic mobility of the M components was evaluated according to the schematic drawing presented in Figure 1.

On Figure 3 some of the most often appearing immunoelectrophoretic abnormalities in MS patients are demonstrated. Besides the abnormalities in the IgG and the IgA precipitate and the presence of the IgM precipitation arc in the CSF immunoelectropherogram, a cathodal elongation and increased density of the cathodal segment of the CSF albumin precipitate (classification 1-C)[38] can be noted. In addition, a cathodal displacement of the hemopexin precipitation arc is seen. An example of an abnormal "shadow" formation in the middle segment of the IgG precipitate showing the corresponding electrophoretic mobility in the

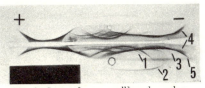

Fig. 3. Serum [upper well] and cerebrospinal fluid immunoelectropherograms. In the middle groove antihuman rabbit antiserum and in the lateral grooves an anti-IgA rabbit antiserum were used. Presence of the IgM precipitate (1), cathodal elongation of the IgA precipitation arc (2), cathodal displacement of the hemopexin precipitate (3) and the gamma-E fraction (5) is demonstrated in the cerebrospinal fluid immunoelectropherogram. A split in the cathodal segment of the serum and cerebrospinal fluid IgG precipitate (4) is suspected. In addition, the albumin precipitate exhibits increased density and elongation of its cathodal segment.

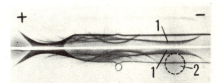

Fig. 4. Serum [upper well] and cerebrospinal fluid immunoelectropherograms. In the middle groove antihuman rabbit antiserum and in the lateral grooves rabbit antiserum against the Fab fragments of IgG were applied. A "shadow" formation showing corresponding electrophoretic mobility (1) is demonstrated. Abnormal staining patterns (2) in the gamma globulin region are also seen.

151

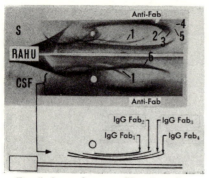

Fig. 5. Serum [upper well] and cerebro-spinal fluid immunoelectropherograms. In the middle groove rabbit antihuman antiserum (RAHU) and in the lateral grooves rabbit antiserum against Fab fragments of IgG were used. The serum IgM precipitate (1) shows "shadow" formation. The IgM pre-cipitation arc is also demonstrated in the cerebrospinal fluid immunoelectropherogram (1). Four precipitation arcs (2-3-4-5) ex-hibiting almost identical electrophoretic mo-bility and configuration in the serum and cerebrospinal fluid immunoelectrophero-grams are schematically drawn in the lower portion of the figure. A definite "shadow" formation in the spinal fluid IgG precipitate (6) is also seen.

serum and CSF immunoelectropherograms is presented in Figure 4. The same figure also shows abnormal staining patterns and the gam-ma-E fraction in the CSF immunoelectrophero-gram. "Fuzziness" in Figure 3 in the cathodal ends of the serum and CSF IgG precipitates usually indicates abnormalities which may be better demonstrated using antiserum against the anti-Fab fragments of IgG. More detailed studies regarding the pathological manifesta-tions in the cathodal segment of the precipi-tates of Fab fragments of IgG will be present-ed elsewhere.[19] Appearance of four precipita-tion arcs using the anti-Fab fragments anti-serum in the serum and CSF is demonstrated in Figure 5. Noteworthy is the almost identi-cal position and configuration of the serum and CSF precipitates, mainly in the cathodal seg-ment. In addition, a "shadow" formation in the serum IgM precipitate is also seen.

In 16 MS patients from our series, CSF was immunochemically and immunoelectrophoreti-cally examined using anti-IgD antiserum. In these CSF specimens, IgD was not detected. Serum and CSF were also immunochemically and immunoelectrophoretically studied with anti-kappa and anti-lambda light polypeptide chains antiserums in 15 of our 64 MS patients. The results of these observations are shortly reported elsewhere.[39]

The most often detected abnormalities in the series of our 64 MS patients studied were immunoelectrophoretic abnormalities in the CSF IgG precipitate (80.9%), increased CSF gamma globulin level to over 12% of the total protein concentration (79.3%), elevated CSF IgG level over 4 mg. per 100 ml. (77.7%), CSF gamma to beta globulin ratio mounted over 1 (76.1%), appearance of M components in the CSF gamma globulin region (68.8%), paren-chymal type of the colloidal gold reaction (66.6%), and presence of plasma cells in the CSF cytograms (54%). In our series of MS patients, the highest rate of abnormal findings was obtained when the elevated CSF IgG concentration over 4 mg. per 100 ml. and the immunoelectrophoretic abnormalities in the CSF IgG precipitate were considered together (95.1%).

DISCUSSION

The high proportion of our MS patients showing elevated CSF IgG concentration and increased amount of the CSF gamma globulins indicates a local production or accumulation or both of IgG or gamma globulins or both in the CNS structures.

However, over 33% of the MS patients stud-ied exhibit abnormal concentration in one or more of the serum immunoglobulins. In addi-tion, in over 20% of the MS patients, one or two M components in the serum gamma globu-lin region showed corresponding electrophoret-ic mobility with M components in the CSF gamma globulin field. In 29.6% of the MS pa-tients studied, immunoelectrophoretic abnor-malities in the IgG precipitation arc or in the precipitate of the Fab fragments of IgG or both displayed corresponding electrophoretic mobility and configuration of the precipitation lines in the serum and CSF immunoelectro-pherograms. The presence of three to four precipitation arcs produced in serum and CSF with the anti-Fab fragments antiserum (Fig.

5) is highly suggestive of an abnormal hyperproduction of IgG subclasses or IgG paraproteins or both. Very similar precipitation arcs in the serum IgG precipitate produced with the polyvalent human antiserum can also be demonstrated in SSPE.[19] Elevation or abnormal decrease in the serum IgA or IgM concentration or both was found in 26.2% of our MS patients. In the CSF specimens the quantitative abnormalities in the IgA or IgM levels or both were found in 46% of the patients. There was no significant relation between the abnormal concentrations of serum and CSF immunoglobulins. With the exception of one patient in our series of MS cases who suffered from widespread decubiti, no clinical signs of chronic irritation of extraneural lymphoreticular structures were noted. In addition, no correlations were found between the abnormal concentrations of serum immunoglobulins and the elevated white blood cell counts or abnormal findings in urine or both. It is highly improbable that the pathological findings in serum gamma globulins in our MS patients merely reflect the proteosynthetic activity of the immunocompetent cells in the CNS structures. In the course of MS the extraneural lymphoreticular tissues also appear to be activated, probably during certain phases of the pathological process.

Regarding the studies of Lowenthal et al.,[18] Cutler et al.,[28] and Kolar[27,29] in SSPE, the qualitative abnormalities in serum gamma globulins of our MS cases indicate that the gamma globulins accumulated in the CNS structures of MS patients are not completely disintegrated locally by macrophages and astrocytes[40] but may pass the blood-brain barrier into the bloodstream. The immunopathological implications of this phenomenon in respect to the pathogenesis of chronic inflammatory or demyelinating CNS afflictions or both are poorly understood. In addition to the proteosynthetic activity occurring in the CNS of MS patients, a certain proportion of gamma globulins produced in extraneural lymphoreticular structures probably penetrates the blood-CNS barrier, a fact demonstrated, for example, in patients with multiple myeloma.[5,19]

In one of our MS cases in whom the serum and CSF specimens were obtained during a regressive phase of the neurological symptomatology and in one 70-year-old patient, no definite abnormalities in the serum and CSF immunoglobulins could be found. Otherwise, in the MS patients, there were no significant correlations established between the phase and extent of the clinical symptomatology and the abnormal serum and CSF findings.

Using antihemopexin antiserum, a cathodal displacement of the CSF hemopexin precipitate was demonstrated in 18.1% of the MS patients studied. This abnormality could be misinterpreted in some instances as a gamma-E fraction.

The authors are indebted to Dr. Charles Spurgeon for the assistance in assembling clinical data; to Miss M. O'Connel, Miss C. Aleyea, and Mrs. D. Albright for technical assistance; to Mrs. E. Solow (Department of Neurosurgery) for the ultraviolet spectrophotometric determination of total proteins; to Mr. J. Glore for drawing; and to Mr. J. Demma for photography.

REFERENCES

1. KABAT, E. A., MOORE, D. H., and LANDOW, H.: An electrophoretic study of the protein components in cerebrospinal fluid and their relationship to the serum proteins. J. clin. Invest. 21:517, 1942.
2. TOURTELLOTTE, W. W., and PARKER, J. A.: Multiple sclerosis: Correlation between immunoglobulin-G in cerebrospinal fluid and brain. Science 154:1044, 1966.
3. SIMPSON, J. F., TOURTELLOTTE, W. W., KOKMEN, E., PARKER, J. A., and ITABASHI, H. H.: Fluorescent protein tracing in multiple sclerosis brain tissue. Arch. Neurol. (Chic.) 20:373, 1969.
4. KOLAR, O., DENCKER, S. J., OBRUCNIK, M., CERNA, I., and SKATULA, Z.: Zur Bedeutung der G-Globulinfraktion im Hirngewebe bei der subakuten sklerotisierenden Leukoencephalitis. Dtsch. Z. Nervenheilk. 188:222, 1966.
5. GERSTL, B., UYEDA, C. T., ENG, L. E., BOND, P., and SMITH, J. K.: Soluble proteins in normal and diseased human brains. Neurology (Minneap.) 19:1019, 1969.
6. YAHR, M. D., GOLDENSOHN, S. S., and KABAT, E. A.: Further studies on the gamma globulin content of cerebrospinal fluid in multiple sclerosis and other neurological diseases. Ann. N.Y. Acad. Sci. 58:613, 1954.
7. HARTLEY, T. F., MERRILL, D. A., and CLAMAN, H. N.: Quantitation of immunoglobulins in cerebrospinal fluid. Arch. Neurol. (Chic.) 15:472, 1966.
8. SCHNECK, S. A., and CLAMAN, H. N.: CSF immunoglobulins in multiple sclerosis and other neurologic diseases. Arch. Neurol. (Chic.) 20:132, 1969.
9. PUTNAM, F. W.: Immunoglobulin structure: Variability and homology. Science 163:633, 1969.
10. COHEN, S., and BANNISTER, R.: Immunoglobulin synthesis within the central nervous system in the disseminated sclerosis. Lancet 1:366, 1967.
11. SANDBERG-WOLLHEIM, M., ZETTERVAL, O., and MULLER, R.: In vitro synthesis of IgG by cells from the cerebrospinal fluid in a patient with multiple sclerosis. Clin. exp. Immunol. 4:401, 1969.
12. ZETTERVAL, O., and LINK, H.: The light chain types of immunoglobulin in CSF. Abstract of paper, Ninth Internat. Congr. Neurol. Exerpta med. 193:303, 1969.
13. GRIMM, R., ALTER, M., and WILLIAMS, R. D.: Gm and Inv antigenic character of serum and cerebrospinal fluid IgG in multiple sclerosis. Proc. Soc. exp. Med. 122:554, 1966.
14. BERG, O., and KALLEN, B.: Effect of mononuclear cells from multiple sclerosis patients on neuroglia in tissue culture. J. Neuropath. exp. Neurol. 23:550, 1964.
15. LOWENTHAL, A., VAN SANDE, M., and KARCHER, D.: The differential diagnosis of neurological diseases by

fractionating electrophoretically the CSF gamma-globulins. J. Neurochem. 6:51, 1960.

16. LATERRE, E. D.: L'électrophorèse en agar des protéines du liquide cephalorachidien. Semiologie de la zone gamma. Acta neurol. belg. 66:289, 1966.

17. FADILOGLU, M.: Les gammaglobulines du serum et de liquide céphalorachidien dans la leucoencéphalite sclérosante subaigue et la sclérose en plaques. Acta neurol. belg. 67:736, 1967.

18. LOWENTHAL, A., KARCHER, D., and VAN SANDE, M.: Analyse électrophorètique des protéines seriques dans la leucoencephalite sclérosante subaiguë. Livre jubilaire Docteur Ludo van Bogaert. Acta neurol. belg. 62:506, 1962.

19. KOLAR, O., MATHEWS, F., HERMAN, J., and MANN, D.: M-components in the gamma-globulin region of CSF electropherograms: Diagnostic aspects. In preparation.

20. DENCKER, S. J.: Immunoelectrophoretic investigation of cerebrospinal fluid gamma-globulins in multiple sclerosis. Acta neurol. scand. 40(suppl. 10):57, 1964.

21. ZEGERS, B. J.: Une micro-méthode de l'immuno-électrophorèse. Int. Arch. Allergy 7:103, 1955.

22. BAUER, H. J., GOTTESLEBEN, A., and WARECKA, K.: Quantitative Immunochemie der Liquor proteine. In: Zukunft der Neurologie. Edited by H. D. Bamme and P. Vogel. Stuttgart: George Thieme Verlag, 1967, p. 200.

23. ZEGERS, B. J., POEN, H., STOOP, J. W., and BALLIEUX, R. E.: Immunoglobulin determination. Evaluation of the results of immunoelectrophoretic analysis and the radial diffusion method. Clin. chim. Acta 22:399, 1968.

24. ENGEL, R., and FRANK, A.: Die Immunoelektrophorese in der Differentialdiagnose paraproteinämischer Erkrankungen. Dtsch. med. Wschr. 90:1281, 1965.

25. SZABO, S.: Recherches biochimiques et immunologiques dans la sclérose en plaques. Acta neurol. belg. 68:682, 1968.

26. CLAUSEN, J.: Immunoelectrophoretic investigations of normal and pathologic cerebrospinal fluid. Wld Neurol. 1:479, 1960.

27. KOLAR, O.: Zur Bedeutung der pathologischen Protein-komponenten im Liquor cerebrospinalis und im Serum von Patienten mit der subakuten Encephalitis nach Dawson-Pette-Döring-van Bogaert. Klin. Wschr. 44:279, 1966.

28. CUTLER, R. W. P., WATTERS, G. V., HAMMERSTAD, J.

P., and MERLER, E.: Origin of cerebrospinal fluid gamma globulin in subacute sclerosing leukoencephalitis. Arch. Neurol. (Chic.) 17:620, 1967.

29. KOLAR, O., and ZEMAN, W.: Immunoelectrophoretic changes of serum IgG during subacute inflammatory and demyelinating diseases of the central nervous system. Z. Immun.-Forsch. 134:267, 1967.

30. KOLAR, O.: Problems of the origin of the anodic part of celebrospinal fluid gamma-G-globulins in inflammatory affections of the central nervous system. Nature (Lond.) 214:524, 1967.

31. KOLAR, O.: Serum Fab-fragment in multiple sclerosis and subacute sclerosing panencephalitis. Lancet 1:1041, 1968.

32. BERGMANN, L., DENCKER, S. J., JOHANSSON, B. G., and SVENNERHOLDM, L.: Cerebrospinal fluid gamma-globulin in subacute sclerosing leucoencephalitis. J. Neurochem. 15:781, 1968.

33. MERRILL, D., HARTLEY, T., and CLAMAN, H.: Electroimmunodiffusion (EID): A single, rapid method for quantitation of immunoglobulins in diluted biological fluids. J. Lab. clin. Med. 69:151, 1967.

34. KOLAR, O.: Fab fragments in central nervous system disorders. Z. Immun.-Forsch. 136:392, 1968.

35. WADELL, W. J., and HILL, C.: A simple ultraviolet spectrophotometric method for the determination of protein. J. Lab. clin. Med. 52:311, 1956.

36. HARTLEY, T. F., MERRILL, D. A., and CLAMAN, H. N.: Quantitation of immunoglobulins in cerebrospinal fluid. Arch. Neurol. (Chic.) 15:472, 1966.

37. KOLAR, O., and ZEMAN, W.: Spinal fluid cytomorphology. Arch. Neurol. (Chic.) 18:44, 1968.

38. KOLAR, O. J., ROSS, A. T., and HERMAN, J. T.: Paraalbumins in cerebrospinal fluid. Neurology (Minneap.) 19:826, 1969.

39. KOLAR, O., and DICKINSON, E.: Comments to the problems of the origin and significance of immunoglobulins in multiple sclerosis. In: Immunological Disorders of the Nervous System. 49th Annual Meeting of the Association for Research in Nervous and Mental Disease, New York, 1969. In press.

40. BLAKEMORE, W. F.: The fate of escaped plasma protein after thermal necrosis of the rat brain: an electron-microscopic study. J. Neuropath. exp. Neurol. 28:139, 1969.

154

Bengt Källén
Olle Nilsson

Mixed Leucocyte Reaction in Multiple Sclerosis

Astorga and Williams[1] have demonstrated that leucocytes from some patients with rheumatoid arthritis (RA) have an impaired one-way mixed leucocyte reaction[2] (MLR) when stimulated with leucocytes from other such patients. No definite explanation of this phenomenon is given. We have investigated other diseases in which auto-immune aetiology is suspected to see whether similar phenomena are associated with them. Here we report our investigations of multiple sclerosis (MS).

The MLR was carried out with peripheral blood leucocytes from fourteen MS patients and from ten patients with various other neurological diseases (non-MS patients). None of the patients were given any drug that might influence the MLR. Cells from each patient were tested against those of another patient with the same diagnosis and with cells from one and the same control person, with HL-A antigens 1, Li, and LND. In each test, cells from one individual were pretreated for 20 min at 37° C with 25 μg/ml. of mito-mycin C (Sigma) and then washed twice with Parker 199 by centrifugation. Leucocytes were separated with dextran and cultured in a medium made up of 30% human blood donor serum, 70% Parker 199, heparin and antibiotics[3]. The cell concentration was 10^6 cells/ml. in each case and the culture time was 7 days. In each case the following combinations were tested : (1) untreated control cells + mitomycin-treated patient cells; (2) untreated patient cells + mitomycin-treated control cells; (3) untreated patient cells + mitomycin-treated cells from another patient of the same diagnosis group. For each group 1.5 ml. of culture was placed in a culture tube. Cells from one tube were stained with acetic orcein[3] to study cell survival. Cells in the other three tubes were labelled with 1 μCi/ml. of methyl-^{3}H-thymidine (Schwarz BioResearch, specific activity 1.9 Ci/mM) for 1 h, washed once with Parker 199, extracted for 30 min with cold 5% trichloroacetic acid (TCA), washed once with cold TCA and once with absolute alcohol. The residue was dissolved in 1 ml. of 1 M NaOH for 1 h at 37° C. A sample (0.1 ml.) of this solution was mixed with 1 ml. of Soluene (Packard Ltd) and 14 ml. of scintillation mixture

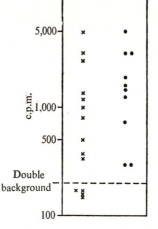

Fig. 1 C.p.m. on a logarithmic scale in patient–patient combinations. ×, MS patients; ●, non-MS patients.

(300 mg dimethyl-POPOP, 5 mg PPO, 1,000 ml. toluene). The radioactivity of the samples was assayed in a Packard Tri-Carb 3310 liquid scintillator and expressed as c.p.m.

Fig. 1 gives the c.p.m., on a logarithmic scale, of patient–patient pairs. Of the ten non-MS patients, all had counts above double background level; of the fourteen MS patients, four showed no response—their c.p.m. were below the double background. This difference is perhaps random, but in this comparison the control combinations which might give further information about the responding and stimulating capacity of cells from each individual were not considered.

The data were analysed as follows : for each group of three identically treated tubes, the arithmetic mean of the logarithms of their radioactivity was calculated. For each patient, three differences between such group means were calculated. *A*, The mean log of c.p.m. was calculated for the combination of control cells + mitomycin-treated patient cells minus mean log of c.p.m. for the combination of the same patient cells + mitomycin-treated control cells. *B*, The mean log of c.p.m. was calculated for the combination of cells from patient "one" + mitomycin-treated control cells minus log of c.p.m. for the combination of cells from patient "one" + mitomycin-treated cells from patient "two" (patients "one" and "two" belong to the same diagnosis group). *C*, The mean log of c.p.m. was calculated for the combination of control cells + mitomycin-treated cells from patient "one" minus mean log of c.p.m. for the combination of cells from patient "two" + mitomycin-

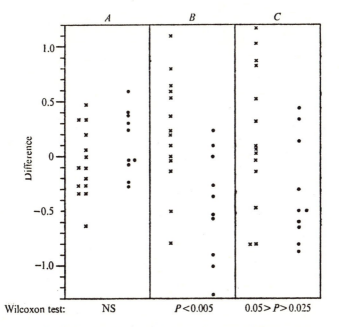

Fig. 2 Differences in log of c.p.m. in three different combinations. *A*, *B*, and *C* are explained in the text. ×, MS patients; ●, non-MS patients.

treated cells from patient "one". *A*, Estimated possible differences in capacity of stimulation in control–patient pairs; *B*, estimated possible differences in the capacity of patient cells to be stimulated by cells from the control and from another patient from the same diagnosis group; and *C*, estimated possible differences in the capacity of patient cells to stimulate cells from the control or from another patient from the same diagnosis group. If the results from patients with rheumatoid arthritis are similar to those from MS patients, *A* should be the same for both MS and non-MS patients, but *B* and *C* should differ.

Fig. 2 presents the results of these calculations. Statistical significance was tested by the Wilcoxon rank test. *A* was the same for both groups; *B* differed significantly; *C* was probably significantly different. Fig. 2 reveals that the cells from some MS patients responded less well than expected in MLR when combined with mitomycin-treated MS cells. In this respect, multiple sclerosis is similar to rheumatoid arthritis.

This work was supported by grants from the Swedish Medical Research Council and the Swedish Cancer Society. We thank Dr Bengt Löw for HL-A typing the control subject.

[1] Astorga, G. P., and Williams, jun., R. C., *Arthrit. Rheum.*, **12**, 547 (1969).
[2] Bach, F. H., and Voynow, N. K., *Science*, **153**, 545 (1966).
[3] Källén, B., and Levan, A., *Cytogenetics* (Basel), **1**, 5 (1962).

IMPAIRED MIXED LEUCOCYTE REACTION IN SOME DIFFERENT DISEASES, NOTABLY MULTIPLE SCLEROSIS AND VARIOUS ARTHRITIDES

HELGE HEDBERG, B. KÄLLÉN, B. LÖW AND O. NILSSON

INTRODUCTION

A blast transformation, accompanied by DNA synthesis and eventually mitosis, occurs when leucocytes from genetically non-identical individuals are mixed in tissue cultures, the so-called mixed leucocyte reaction or MLR (Bain, Vas & Lowenstein, 1964, cf. review by Ling, 1968). The strength of the response depends on the number of differences in HL-A antigens present in the combination (Schellekens *et al.*, 1970). A reaction occurs, however, between cells from unrelated donors also at identical HL-A antigens (Kissmeyer-Nielsen *et al.*, 1970).

Reactions will, in most instances, be obtained in MLR between genetically dissimilar individuals. Experimentally induced tolerance in rats prevents the reaction (Wilson, Silvers & Nowell, 1967; Schwarz, 1968); treatment with antilymphocytic serum extinguishes it (Greaves *et al.*, 1967; Hardy & Ling, 1969). Leucocytes from pregnant women have been said to show no, or only poor, response to their husband's leucocytes despite a normal response to leucocytes from other men (Lewis *et al.*, 1966; Halbrecht & Komlos, 1968). This was explained as being due to a state of specific tolerance induced by the conceptus. Astorga & Williams (1969) demonstrated that leucocytes from some patients with rheumatoid arthritis (RA) showed an impaired MLR when stimulated with leucocytes from other RA patients. Källén & Nilsson (1971) found similar conditions in patients with multiple sclerosis (MS). These findings have been further extended in the present study to comprise also other disease groups.

MATERIALS AND METHODS

MLR was performed with peripheral blood leucocytes from twenty-four control individuals (twelve patients with neurological diseases other than MS and twelve healthy individuals), from eighteen patients with MS, twelve patients with RA, twenty-eight patients with other diseases (two with SLE, two with scleroderma, twelve with psoriasis arthropatica, and twelve with pelvospondylitis). Each subject was tested in one-way MLR against another subject and against a healthy person, who will be called 'standard' in order to distinguish him from the controls just mentioned. Three standards were used. The HL-A types of these three persons were: HL-A 1, Li, and LND; 1 and 8; 1, Ba, 8, and 12.

Leucocytes were separated from heparinized blood with 6% dextran (Macrodex, Pharmacia), 2·5 ml dextran per 10 ml blood. The tube was left in a slanting position for 30–45 min until erythrocytes had sedimented. The leucocytes were then spun down and suspended to a cell concentration of 2×10^6 cells/ml in a medium consisting of 30% heat inactivated adult human blood donor serum and 70% Parker 199 (SBL, Stockholm), and containing heparin and antibiotics. Half the portion of the cell suspension was pretreated for 20 min at 37°C with mitomycin C (Sigma) 25 μg/ml (Bach & Voynow, 1966), and then washed twice with Parker 199. In the one-way reaction tests, the cells from one individual were thus pretreated (stimulating cells), those from the other individual were not pretreated (reacting cells).

Individuals were tested in pairs, the members of a pair usually belonged to the same diagnostic group. If P_1 and P_2 = two such individuals, S = the used standard, and -mit = pre-treatment of the cell population with mitomycin (cf. Fig. 1), the following combinations were performed: ($P_1 + P_2$-mit), (P_1-mit + P_2), (P_1-mit + S), (P_1 + S-mit), (P_2-mit + S), (P_2 + S-mit).

In each of these six combinations, three identical cultures were set up, each with 1·5 ml of cell suspension, half of which thus came from each member of the pair. The tubes were incubated at 37°C for 7 days and then labelled with 1 μCi/ml of methyl-[³H]thymidine (Schwarz BioResearch Inc., spec. act. 1·9 Ci/mM) for 1 hr, then washed once with Parker 199, extracted for 30 min with cold 5% TCA, washed once with cold TCA and once with absolute alcohol. The residue was then dissolved in 1 ml of 1 N NaOH for 1 hr at 37°. 0·1 ml of this solution was mixed with 1 ml of Soluene (Packard Ltd) and 14 ml of scintillation mixture (300 mg dimethyl-POPOP, 5 mg PPO, 1000 ml toluene). The radioactivity of the samples was assayed in a Packard TriCarb 3310 liquid scintillator and expressed as counts/min. Background activity was determined from a blank, and this value was subtracted from the registered counts/min. Counting was made during two 10 min periods.

Because of technical faults, no uptake was registered in any combination in a few experiments, which were therefore excluded.

160

Twenty-four MLRs were performed between controls. In all, an activity well above double background was registered. Each except one of these controls was also tested against a standard. Of twenty-three 'control + standard-mit' combinations, two showed an uptake near double background, and of twenty-three 'control-mit + standard' combinations one did so. Of seventy random combinations in the control material, thus three lacked a clear-cut MLR response. This is most probably due to technical faults.

In the patient–patient combinations, nineteen out of fifty-six showed non-significant MLR (activity below double background). Compared with the frequency found among the controls (three out of seventy), the difference is highly significant ($\chi^2 = 19\cdot0$, $P < 0\cdot001$). Of these nineteen tests, five were made with MS patients and three with RA patients. Eleven are found in twenty-eight patients with one of the diagnoses: psoriasis arthropatica, SLE, scleroderma, or pelvospondylitis ($\chi^2 = 20\cdot0$, $P < 0\cdot001$). When the frequencies found in the groups of psoriasis arthropatica or pelvospondylitis (five out of twelve in each) are tested against the control frequency, Fisher's exact test gives $P = 0\cdot0013$. Each of these two groups is thus in itself highly significantly different from the controls. Of fifty-five patient + standard-mit combinations, two showed a lack of response, and of fifty-five patient-mit + standard combinations, another one did not respond. These frequencies do not differ from that found in the control material (three out of seventy).

The calculations so far have only taken into account MLRs without any significant thymidine incorporation. In some instances, there was a significant thymidine uptake in the patient–patient MLR, but this uptake was markedly below that in the patient–standard combinations. This can be exemplified by the SLE pair (Table 2).

Cells from patient SLE 1 thus react with a thymidine uptake of 2·87 (expressed as mean log counts/min values) when responding to cells from patient SLE 2, but with 3·50 (over four times more) when responding to standard cells. Similarly, SLE 1 cells when stimulating SLE 2 cells induced an uptake of 2·60 only, but of 3·24 when stimulating standard cells (also over four times more). To estimate the MLR capacities of this patient's cells (SLE 1) the differences between the logarithms can be used: the capacity to respond is thus estimated by the difference 0·63, and the capacity to stimulate by the difference 0·64. Now, in these differences will also enter (besides random variations) differences due to the degree of similarities in transplantation antigens between the patients and between the patient and the standard. The log differences must therefore be compared between groups of patients and controls. This has been done with the use of the two above-mentioned differences, supplemented by a third, which is included as a check on the responsiveness of the cells; namely, the difference between the uptake in standard cells when stimulated with patient cells and the uptake of patient cells when stimulated with standard cells.

Thus, three characteristics will be given for each patient (cf. Fig. 1):

A: Mean log counts/min for combination $S + P_1$-mit *minus* mean log counts/min for combination S-mit $+ P_1$: this estimates possible differences in responsiveness between patient and standard cells.

B: Mean log of counts/min for S-mit $+ P_1$ *minus* the same for P_2-mit $+ P_1$: this estimates possible differences in the capacity of patient cells to be stimulated by cells from the standard and from another patient.

161

TABLE 1. Frequency of one-way MLR tests without significant thymidine uptake (below double background) in different combinations of individuals; denominators = total number of patients studied

Cell source		Frequency of non-significant thymidine uptake
Reacting cells	Mitomycin-pretreated cells	
I. Combinations of patient–patient		
MS	MS	5/18
RA	RA	3/10
Psoriasis arthropatica	Psoriasis arthropatica	5/12
Pelvospondylitis	Pelvospondylitis	5/12
SLE	SLE	0/2
Scleroderma	Scleroderma	1/2
		Total: 19/56
II. Combination of patient–standard		
MS	Standard	0/18
RA	Standard	1/10
Psoriasis arthropatica	Standard	0/11
Pelvospondylitis	Standard	1/12
SLE	Standard	0/2
Sclerodermia	Standard	0/2
		Total: 2/55
Standard	MS	0/18
Standard	RA	0/10
Standard	Psoriasis arthropatica	0/11
Standard	Pelvospondylitis	1/12
Standard	SLE	0/2
Standard	Sclerodermia	0/2
		Total: 1/55

TABLE 2. Response in MLR between two patients with SLE and a standard

Cell source		Mean log of counts/min above background
Reacting cells	Mitomycin-pretreated cells	
SLE 1	SLE 2	2·87
SLE 2	SLE 1	2·60
SLE 1	Standard	3·50
SLE 2	Standard	2·90
Standard	SLE 1	3.24
Standard	SLE 2	2·77

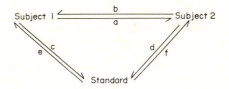

FIG. 1. Diagram showing the one-way MLR tests performed. a–f, represent log counts/min values in the one-way reactions with the direction indicated by the arrows. The following calculations are made:

	Subject 1	Subject 2
A	c–e	d–f
B	e–b	f–a
C	c–a	d–b

TABLE 3. Results of comparisons of differences A–C (see text) between groups of subjects

Difference studied	Patient group	No. of tests	Mean ± S.E.M.	Comparison with controls			
				Student's test		Wilcoxon's test	
				t	P	T^*	P
A	Controls	23	0.171 ± 0.081	—	—	—	—
	MS	18	-0.011 ± 0.107	1·38	0·2–0·1	342	>0·1
	RA	10	-0.007 ± 0.120	1·65	0·2–0·1	135	>0·1
	Pelvospondylitis	12	-0.044 ± 0.101	1·61	0·2–0·1	174	>0·1
	Psoriasis arthropatica	12	-0.021 ± 0.109	1·40	0·2–0·1	185·5	>0·1
B	Controls	23	-0.406 ± 0.116	—	—	—	—
	MS	18	0.182 ± 0.126	3·42	0·005–0·001	494	<0·01
	RA	10	0.482 ± 0.147	4·42	<0·001	264·5	<0·01
	Pelvospondylitis	12	0.488 ± 0.136	4·75	<0·001	327·5	<0·01
	Psoriasis arthropatica	12	0.570 ± 0.171	4·83	<0·001	326	<0·01
C	Controls	23	-0.227 ± 0.086	—	—	—	—
	MS	18	0.092 ± 0.125	2·51	0·02–0·01	463·5	0·05–0·02
	RA	10	0.381 ± 0.169	3·84	<0·001	253	<0·01
	Pelvospondylitis	12	0.444 ± 0.111	5·01	<0·001	330	<0·01
	Psoriasis arthropatica	12	0.506 ± 0.161	4·71	<0·001	320·5	<0·01

* T value refers to the patient group.

C: Mean log of counts/min for combination $S + P_1$-mit *minus* the same for $P_2 + P_1$-mit: this estimates the possible differences in the capacity to stimulate standard cells and cells from another patient.

163

Table 3 gives mean values with standard errors of the means for controls and for four groups of patients. The different groups are compared with t-tests and Wilcoxon's tests— the latter test was used to ensure that a non-normal distribution of the differences A – C could not markedly interfere with the conclusions drawn.

All groups show similar means with respect to the difference A. Thus there are no indications that the patient cells *per se* were poor responders in an MLR against a healthy person (standard).

In the B differences, significantly higher values were found in all four groups of patients. This means that, on average, patients of these groups respond less than controls in an MLR when stimulated by another patient with the same diagnosis. Similarly, the mean C differences are higher in all patient groups, showing that patient cells are also poor stimulators.

It is noteworthy that both B and C means for controls are significantly below zero. This would mean that the standard cells used are poorer moitiers in MLR than the average control cells. The explanation of this is unclear. It might be due to the antigen composition or to technical factors. A variance analysis reveals no difference either in A, B, or C values between the control combinations with the three standards used.

DISCUSSION

The observation published by Astorga & Williams (1969) that cells from RA patients do not react as well with each other in an MLR as with control cells is verified in the present study. This study also shows that this phenomenon is not restricted to RA patients but applies also to patients with some other diseases. A common feature of most of these diseases is that an immunological component has been implied in their pathogenesis. This is true for MS and RA, SLE, and scleroderma. Psoriasis arthropatica was shown to have similarities with SLE with respect to the cytolytic activity of lymphoid cells removed from the inflamed joint (Hedberg, 1967).

The explanation of the phenomenon of impaired MLR in these diseases is unclear. Twomey *et al.* (1970) pointed out that, in order to get an MLR, the following criteria must be fulfilled besides the obviously necessary difference in antigen composition mentioned in the introduction; (a) mitotically responsive lymphocytes must be present, (b) a sufficient quantity of allogenic cells must be present, (c) at least 1 % of functionally intact macrophages must be present in either the reacting or the stimulating cell population, and (d) culture time must be optimum (usually 5–7 days).

There is no reason to believe that the distribution of HL-A antigens differs so much in patients with the various diseases and the controls as to explain the lack of MLR response. To check this, HL-A antigen composition was determined in four pairs without MLR. None of the pairs showed a complete HL-A match. It is theoretically possible that the antigenic composition of the lymphocytes is somehow masked. However, the cells react with standard cells. For the same reason, the mitotic responsiveness of the lymphocytes is obviously not impaired.

No reduction in macrophage numbers is known to occur in these diseases, but an impaired macrophage function is one possible explanation of the poor MLR. As it does not matter whether the macrophages belong to the stimulating or the responding population, this would explain why normal MLRs are obtained with the standard cells. Further studies along this line are planned as are also studies of the time factor.

ACKNOWLEDGMENT

The costs of this investigation were defrayed by grants from the Swedish Cancer Society (Project No. 108-B70), The Swedish Multiple Sclerosis Foundation and from the immunological research fund of Astra Corp., Södertälje, Sweden.

REFERENCES

ASTORGA, G.P. & WILLIAMS, R.C., JR (1969) Altered reactivity in mixed lymphocyte culture of lymphocytes from patients with rheumatoid arthritis. *Arthr. and Rheum.* **12**, 547.

BACH, F. & VOYNOW, N.K. (1966) One-way stimulation in mixed leukocyte culture. *Science*, **153**, 545.

BAIN, B., VAS, M.R. & LOWENSTEIN, L. (1964) The development of large immature mononuclear cells in mixed lymphocyte cultures. *Blood*, **23**, 108.

GREAVES, M., ROITT, I.M., ZAMIR, R. & CARNAGHAN, R.B.A. (1967) Effect of antilymphocyte serum on response of human peripheral-blood lymphocytes to specific and non-specific stimulants in vitro. *Lancet*, **ii**, 1317.

HALBRECHT, I. & KOMLOS, L. (1968) Lymphocyte transformation in mixed wife–husband leukocyte culture in abortions and in hydatidiform moles. *Obstet. and Gynec.* **31**, 173.

HARDY, D.A. & LING, N.R. (1969) Effects of some cellular antigens on lymphocytes and the nature of the mixed lymphocyte reaction. *Nature (Lond.)* **221**, 554.

HEDBERG, H. (1967) Studies on synovial fluid in arthritis. II. The occurrence of mononuclear cells with *in vitro* cytotoxic effect. *Acta med. scand.* (Suppl.) **479**, 79.

KÄLLÉN, B. & NILSSON, O. (1971) Mixed leukocyte reaction in multiple sclerosis. *Nature (Lond.)*, **229**, 91.

KISSMEYER-NIELSEN, F., SVEJGAARD, A., FREIESLEBEN-SØRENSEN, S., STAUB NIELSEN, L. & THORSBY, E. (1970) Mixed lymphocyte culture and HL-A identity in unrelated subjects. *Nature (Lond.)*, **228**, 63.

LEWIS, J., JR, WHANG, J., NAGEL, B., JOOST, B.A., OPPENHEIM, J. & PERRY, S. (1966) Lymphocyte transformation in mixed leukocyte cultures in women with normal pregnancy or tumors of placental origin. *Amer. J. Obstet. Gynec.* **96**, 287.

LING, N.D. (1968) *Lymphocyte stimulation*, North Holland Publ. Co., Amsterdam.

SCHELLEKENS, P.TH.A., VRIESENDORP, B., EIJSVOOGEL, V.P., VAN LEEUWEN, A., VAN ROOD, J.J., MIGGIAND, V. & CEPELLINI, R. (1970) Lymphocyte transformation *in vitro*. II. Mixed lymphocyte culture in relation to leucocyte antigens. *Clin. exp. Immunol.* **6**, 241.

SCHWARZ, M.R. (1968) The mixed lymphocyte reaction: an *in vitro* test for tolerance. *J. exp. Med.* **127**, 879.

TWOMEY, J.J., SHARKEY, O., JR, BROWN, J.A., LAUGHTER, A.H. & JORDAN, P.H., JR (1970) Cellular requirements for the mitotic response in allogeneic mixed leucocyte cultures. *J. Immunol.* **104**, 845.

WILSON, D.B., SILVERS, W.K. & NOWELL, P.C. (1967) Quantitative studies on the mixed lymphocyte interaction in rats. II. Relationship of the proliferative response to the immunologic status of the donors. *J. exp. Med.* **126**, 655.

Lymphocyte Response Depressive Factor in Multiple Sclerosis

E. J. FIELD,   E. A. CASPARY

Introduction

Whatever the aetiology of multiple sclerosis (M.S.) may ultimately turn out to be—infective or autoimmune—it is difficult to escape the conclusion that immunological processes (and delayed hypersensitivity in particular) play a part in the genesis of recurrent episodes of the disease. Since delayed hypersensitivity depends on lymphocyte sensitization and the autoaggression of these cells is believed to produce the disease, any means of damping-down the reactivity of such lymphocytes is of potential therapeutic importance. In the case of M.S. the putative antigen is a basic protein extractable from human brain (Caspary and Field, 1965, 1971a) and capable of producing experimental allergic encephalomyelitis in animals.

In multiple sclerosis (Hughes, Caspary, and Field, 1968; Knowles, Hughes, Caspary, and Field, 1968; van den Noort and Stjernholm, 1971) as well as in a whole variety of other conditions such as tuberculosis (Heilman and McFarland, 1966), hepatitis (Paronetto and Popper, 1970), secondary syphilis (Levene, Turk, Wright, and Grimble, 1969), ataxia telangiectasia (McFarlin and Oppenheim, 1969), and chronic candidiasis (Canales, Middlemas, Louro, and South, 1969) among others, serum has been shown to contain a factor which is able to damp down lymphocytic response to antigen. The present work studies the titre of this lymphocyte depressive factor in normal serum and in serum from patients with M.S. and other (destructive) neurological diseases. The isolation and characterization of the lymphocyte depressive factor might be of considerable therapeutic importance in the treatment of diseases due to "autoaggression" by these cells.

166

Research in human lymphocyte sensitization has hitherto been much hampered by the absence of a sensitive, reproducible, and quantitative method of estimation (Bloom, 1971), but recently we have described one such which we believe has these attributes—the macrophage electrophoretic slowing test (Field and Caspary, 1971b; Caspary and Field, 1971b)—and this has been used in the present work. Its principle is described below.

Patients and Methods

The present work has been carried out exclusively on human serum. (*a*) Four normal subjects have been studied for the depressant effect of autologous and homologous serum—that is, from a different normal—on the interaction of lymphocytes with purified protein derivative of tuberculin (P.P.D.) and measles antigens, two to which there is almost universal lymphocyte sensitization—that is, normal serum has been studied on normal lymphocytes. (*b*) Serum from five normal subjects has been tested for lymphocyte depressive factor on the response of lymphocytes from patients with M.S. and other neurological disease when stimulated with encephalitogenic factor (E.F.), to which they are known to be sensitized (Caspary and Field, 1970). (*c*) Serum from seven cases of chronic M.S. has been tested in the same way for lymphocyte depressive factor on M.S. lymphocytes. (*d*) Serum from five patients with other neurological disease has been tested in the same way for lymphocyte depressive factor on other neurological disease lymphocytes. In addition, the effect of M.S. serum on other neurological disease lymphocytes and vice versa has been examined.

Where serum has been titrated it has been tested at dilutions of 1:60, 1:120, 1:240, and 1:480. Lymphocyte responsiveness to antigen has been assessed throughout by the cell electrophoresis method (as outlined below) which is ordinarily carried out in a balanced salt solution (medium 199).

In principle the method of electrophoretic macrophage slowing depends on the liberation, when antigen meets lymphocyte, of some factor (macrophage slowing factor, which may turn out to be identical with macrophage inhibition factor) with the property of causing normal guinea-pig peritoneal macrophages to travel more slowly in an electric field. For testing normal lymphocytes P.P.D. and measles antigen (grown in LLC MK$_2$ cells) has been used, with the culture alone without virus as control. In all tests with M.S. or other neurological disease patients encephalitogenic basic protein from human brain has been used as antigen. In all cases antigen has been used at a concentration of 33 µg/ml. The interaction between lymphocytes and antigen takes place in medium 199 at 20°C and pH 7·2. A detailed account of the method with full protocol and statistical analysis has been presented elsewhere (Caspary and Field, 1971a) but it must be stressed again that all measurements are made "blind." Briefly, lymphocytes are isolated from about 15 ml of venous blood, using carbonyl iron and methyl cellulose, while peritoneal macrophages are obtained from normal guinea-pigs 8-15 days after intraperitoneal injection of 20 ml of sterile liquid paraffin. The macrophage exudate is exposed to 100 rads of γ-irradiation to eliminate reactivity of the admixed lymphocytes. In carrying out a test 0.5×10^6 lymphocytes are mixed with 10^7 irradiated macrophages in medium 199 and incubated for 90 minutes at 20°C. The macrophage migration time—that is, without antigen—is t_c. To other tubes the antigens to be tested are added and after incubation macrophage migration time is again measured (t_e).

When the effect of serum is to be measured concentrations of 1:60, 1:120, 1:240, and 1:480 are incorporated in the lymphocyte, antigen, and macrophage mixture and the macrophages again timed (t_s).

Results

NORMAL SUBJECTS

In Table I the actual migration times measured, using measles or P.P.D. as antigen, are set out. It will be seen that the increase in time is greatest in the absence of serum—that is, when the test is carried out in medium 199. When serum is present (1:60) in the reacting mixture the prolongation of migration time is less than when it is absent, and this difference is more pronounced with autologous serum than with that from another normal subject. Own serum thus has a more pronounced effect in inhibiting the lymphocyte-antigen interaction than has homologous serum.

TABLE I—*Normal Subjects. Macrophage Migration Time (sec) in Presence of Measles or P.P.D. with and without Serum (1:60)*

Subject No.	Serum	Control (t_c) i.e., No Antigen	Measles Antigen (t_e) No Serum	Measles Antigen + Serum (t_s)	P.P.D. Antigen (t_e) No Serum	P.P.D. Antigen + Serum (t_s)
1	—	5·995*	6·735		7·055	
	1†			6·595		6·855
	2			6·705		7·015
2	—	5·995	6·700		7·100	
	2†			6·620		6·870
	1			6·655		7·020
3	—	6·025	6·700		7·080	
	3†			6·610		6·860
	4			6·680		6·975
4	—	6·015	6·755		7·020	
	4†			6·635		6·840
	3			6·665		6·950

*Each time is calculated as the mean of 20 readings and the S.D. is less than 0·02 sec (full details are given in Caspary and Field, 1971a).
†Autologous serum.

168

The inhibition of lymphocyte response resulting from the incorporation of serum into the test system can be most conveniently expressed by representing the response in medium 199 as 100 and calculating the other results as a proportionate figure. For example in line 1 of Table I, measles antigen causes 6·735-5·995 = 0·740 sec slowing. This is taken as 100. Then in line 2, when autologous serum is present, the slowing is 6·595-5·995 = 0·600 sec and this is represented as 81·1 in line one of Table II. Table II shows the data of Table I presented in this form. Statistical calculation shows that only differences >15·0

TABLE II—*Data of Table I Presented as Described in the Text: 100 Represents Migration Inhibition Result when Test Carried Out in Medium 199*

Subject No.	Serum	Measles	P.P.D.
1	1	81·1	81·1
	2	96·0	96·2
2	2	88·7	79·2
	1	93·6	92·8
3	3	86·7	79·1
	4	97·0	90·0
4	4	83·8	82·1
	3	87·8	93·0

Only a change >15·0 is significant (P <0·01).

are significant (P <0·01). The figures in Tables III-V also represent the calculated values based on 100 as representing the response in absence of serum—that is, in medium 199.

M.S. PATIENTS

The cells of M.S. patients tested with E.F. antigen showed well-marked sensitization to E.F. as reported previously (Caspary and Field, 1970).

(a) The serum of seven M.S. patients (Cases 5-11) was tested for suppressive activity in each case against own lymphocytes and this was compared with the action of homologous serum—that is from a different M.S. patient. As can be seen from Table III, an M.S. serum is much more active against own lymphocytes than is the serum from another patient on those lymphocytes. When P.P.D. is used as the provocate antigen own serum is again more effective than homologous serum—that is, from another case of M.S.

(b) When the lymphocyte-depressing activity of homologous M.S. serum—that is, from other cases of M.S.—was titrated on the cells of three patients (Cases 12, 13, and 14, Table IVa) it can be seen that four of the six homologous sera were active at 1:240. In Case 14 the patient's own serum (autologous) was also titrated out and found to be active to 1:480. Thus M.S. serum was more active on its own cells than were foreign M.S. sera.

169

TABLE III—*M.S. lymphocytes: Suppression Produced by Own Serum (1:60) Compared with that Produced by Sera from Other M.S. Patients (1:60). 100 Represents Migration Inhibition Result when Test Carried Out in Medium 199*

Case No.	Anti-gen	Own	Homologous Serum					
			5	6	7	8	9	16
5 ..	E.F.	58·3	—	—	—	—	—	—
	P.P.D.	61·5	—	—	—	—	—	—
6 ..	E.F.	68·3	—	—	—	83·6	—	—
	P.P.D.	72·2	—	—	—	90·1	—	—
7 ..	E.F.	36·7	—	63·3	—	52·5	67·1	—
	P.P.D.	56·1	—	72·4	—	64·5	69·6	—
8 ..	E.F.	32·9	—	60·3	54·8	—	68·5	—
	P.P.D.	58·6	—	77·7	71·2	—	75·3	—
9 ..	E.F.	32·4	—	64·2	83·8	69·6	—	—
	P.P.D.	61·0	—	80·3	81·7	86·7	—	—
10 ..	E.F.	49·2	—	—	—	68·3	—	—
	P.P.D.	49·6	—	—	—·	65·2	—	—
11 ..	E.F.	40·8	74·6	—	—	—	—	52·7
	P.P.D.	61·7	80·2	—	—	—	—	65·2

Cases 5-11 inclusive and Case 16 suffered from M.S. Case 10 was in an acute phase. Case 11 was subacute.

(*c*) Sera from cases of other neurological disease were titrated out on lymphocytes from M.S. Cases 17 and 18. It can be seen (Table IVb) that depressant activity was preserved to 1:240. Thus other neurological disease serum has the same power to block E.F.-M.S. lymphocyte interaction as has M.S. serum itself.

(*d*) For comparison the blocking ability of normal serum (Cases 1 and 19-22) on E.F.-M.S. lymphocyte interaction was titrated. It is apparent that the activity of normal serum does not extend beyond 1:60.

It is of interest that though Cases 10 and 13 were in an acute phase of M.S. (Tables III and IV) their sera did not show greater blocking activity than those from the other patients who were chronically affected.

TABLE IV—*M.S. Lymphocyte Suppression*

Case No.	Serum	1:60	1:120	1:240	1:480
(a) M.S. lymphocytes; M.S. serum from different patients: E.F. antigen. Inhibitory factor titrated out					
12..	7	53·4	55·6	97·2	97·2
	8	57·9	61·2	66·9	98·9
	9	58·9	59·6	80·3	99·4
13..	15	57·4	66·7	100·6	100·6
	16	58·0	59·3	73·5	101·9
14..	13	59·8	63·4	77·8	96·9
	14	46·4	49·0	58·8	79·4
(b) M.S. lymphocytes; Other Neurological Diseases serum; E.F. antigen					
14..	17	58·2	62·4	77·3	97·4
	18	62·9	61·2	67·5	96·9
(c) M.S. lymphocytes: normal serum: E.F. antigen					
12..	19	84·3	98·3	—	—
	20	86·0	97·2	—	—
	1	80·9	92·6	—	—
13..	21	85·8	98·1	—	—
	22	87·0	98·1	—	—

Cases 5-16 inclusive suffered from M.S. (Cases 10 and 13 were in an acute phase; Case 11 was subacute). Cases 17 and 18 suffered from other neurological diseases Cases 19-22 and Case 1 were healthy normals.
Anything below 85 is P <0·01.

Lymphocytes from patients with destructive neurological disease other than M.S. were sensitized to E.F. in much the same degree as in M.S. (Caspary and Field, 1970). Again serum from such cases depressed the response when introduced into the test system and was active in higher dilution than was normal serum. Just as serum from M.S. patients was active against other neurological disease lymphocytes (Table Vb), serum from other neurological disease patients was active in reducing M.S. lymphocyte reactivity in about equal measure (Table IVb). Similarly the serum of Case 25 (Table Va) was more active against his own cells than was homologous serum. Normal serum (only one specimen tested—Case 32) (Table Vc) had much the same depressant effect on other neurological disease lymphocytes as on M.S. cells—in both cases distinctly less than the disease sera.

TABLE V—*Other Neurological Disease Suppression*

Case No.			Serum	1:60	1:120	1:240	1:480
(a) *Other Neurological Disease lymphocytes; serum from other patients with Other Neurological Disease; E.F. antigen. Inhibitory factor titrated out*							
23..	..	..	28	69·5	66·5	76·8	104·9
			29	61·0	67·1	91·5	99·4
			30	50·9	53·3	65·5	95·2
24..	..	..	31	57·0	59·4	78·8	100·0
			18	57·0	54·5	67·3	98·8
25..	..	..	23	62·2	72·4	80·5	96·2
			25	45·9	57·8	68·6	82·2
(b) *Other Neurological Disease lymphocytes: M.S. serum: E.F. antigen*							
25..	..	..	11	65·4	65·4	81·1	96·8
			15	65·4	68·1	87·6	101·1
26..	..	..	10	—	—	56·8	100·5
(c) *Other Neurological Disease lymphocytes: normal serum: E.F. antigen*							
27..	..	..	32	82·4	98·8	—	—

Cases 23-31 suffered from other neurological diseases. Cases 10, 11, and 15 suffered from M.S. Case 32 was normal.

Discussion

Our results indicate that there is present in the serum of normal subjects and to a greater extent in the serum of patients with destructive neurological disease (including M.S.) a factor which can exert a depressive effect on lymphocyte response to specific antigen as measured by the macrophage slowing technique. Moreover, in the case of normal serum this factor has a greater effect on its own lymphocytes than on those from other normal people. It would thus seem to be "tailor-made" to its own lymphocytes, an example of the "uniqueness of the individual." In patients with M.S. or other neurological disease, serum likewise has a greater effect on autologous lymphocytes than on those from another patient. However, there is no specificity, in that M.S. serum will depress other neurological disease lymphocytes, and other neurological disease serum will depress M.S. lymphocytes. The titre of suppressive activity is clearly greater in sera from patients with M.S. and other neurological disease than in normal serum. We have no evidence that the factor is qualitatively different.

Our finding of lymphocyte responsiveness depressor factor in serum may offer an explanation of a difficulty, not often brought out, which confronts those who attribute to M.S. an essentially autoimmune pathogenesis. It is now clear that sensitization to E.F. occurs as a consequence of brain destruction from any cause and involves both humoral and cellular aspects (Caspary and Field, 1970; Field, Caspary, and Ball, 1963), and indeed appreciable sensitization occurs in a considerable proportion of normal subjects (Field et al., 1963; Caspary and Field, 1970). Why then does M.S. not follow much more frequently as a continuing autoimmune process as a sequel, say, to head injury? Though a number of suggestions might be offered, it seems possible that suppressive factor is produced under such conditions and the development of M.S. might result only from initial or periodic failure of suppressive factor to reach an adequate level. Quantitative serial study of suppressive factor titre over the period of an exacerbation would be important.

We have also established that in other conditions in which lymphocyte sensitization to a variety of antigens has been found —for example sarcoidosis, B.C.G. "non-converters" (Caspary and Field, 1971b)—a serum factor capable of depressing lymphocyte response is also to be found. Indeed the occurrence of such a factor in sarcoidosis, where high lymphocyte sensitization is so commonly accompanied by diminished delayed hypersensitivity skin reactions, is a theoretical necessity. We have found, too, that the newborn child with high lymphocyte sensitivity to P.P.D. (Field and Caspary, 1971a) yet negative Mantoux reaction also has a high level of serum depressive factor.

The inhibitory factor is not specific, in so far as M.S. or sarcoid serum will also interfere with unrelated antigen-lymphocyte interaction. For example, serum (1:60) from a patient with other neurological disease and two M.S. sera reduced a mixed lymphocyte reaction by 23·1, 28·6, and 41·5% respectively. Likewise M.S. serum (1:60) reduced the interaction between bovine serum albumin and lymphocytes in a case of erythema nodosum by 54·8% and for egg albumen by 48·1%. A full account of these studies will be given elsewhere, but it is already clear that the development of lymphocyte sensitization (as indicated by the capacity to interact with a particular antigen) seems to be associated with the appearance in the serum of a depressant factor and that this factor is more effective against its own lymphocytes than those from another individual. In view of the many reports of depressive factor referred to in the introduction, it may be that the present study of M.S. and other neurological disease is but a special instance of a general phenomenon—the simultaneous development of

172

lymphocyte responsiveness and a serum-mediated "damping mechanism." If further studies support this view, then we have another example of a biological "brake-accelerator" mechanism, operating this time in immunological reactivity. The suppressor element might indeed be the "feedback factor" postulated in several modern schemata involving lymphocyte activity—for example, that of Mackler (1971).

It is legitimate to speculate that disease may result from imbalance between lymphocyte reactivity on the one hand and suppressive activity of serum on the other, so that it would be reasonable to attempt therapeutic control of lymphocyte activity (either in positive or negative direction) by increasing or reducing the suppressive factor. Thus autoimmune diseases (if they exist) presumably result from a runaway activity of lymphocytes and might be treated by augmenting the level of suppressor factor. On the other hand, where lymphocyte activity is being held in check physiologically and where its greater exercise might be beneficial—for example, in resistence to cancer—it might be possible to eliminate or reduce suppressor activity. As a first step it is necessary to isolate and characterize the suppressor factor. Its relation to the factor isolated by Cooperband, Bondevik, Schmid, and Mannick (1968) is being explored, but it is already clear that it occurs in the same α2-globulin fraction in normal, M.S., and cancer serum.

We would like to thank Professor J. N. Walton, Dr. D. A. Shaw, and other members of the department of neurology both in the Newcastle General Hospital and in the Royal Victoria Infirmary for allowing us to study patients under their care; and Mrs. J. Cunningham and Mr. A. Keith for help in preparing lymphocytes and macrophages.

The cytopherometers used were provided by the North-East Multiple Sclerosis Society and the Multiple Sclerosis Research Fund Limited.

References

Bloom, B. R. (1971). *New England Journal of Medicine*, 284, 1212.

Canales, L., Middlemas, R. O., Louro, J. M., and South, M. A. (1969). *Lancet*, 2, 567.

Caspary, E. A., and Field, E. J. (1965). *Annals of the New York Academy of Sciences*, 122, 182.

Caspary, E. A., and Field, E. J. (1970). *European Neurology*, 4, 257.

Caspary, E. A., and Field, E. J. (1971a). *British Medical Journal*, 2, 613.

Caspary, E. A., and Field, E. J. (1971b). *British Medical Journal*, 2, 143.

Cooperband, S. R., Bondevik, H., Schmid, K., and Mannick, J. A. (1968). *Science*, 159, 1243.

Field, E. J., Caspary, E. A., and Ball, E. J. (1963). *Lancet*, 2, 11.

Field, E. J., and Caspary, E. A. (1971a). *Lancet*, 2, 337.

Field, E. J., and Caspary, E. A. (1971b). *Journal of Clinical Pathology*, 24, 179.

Heilman, D. H., and McFarland, W. (1966). *International Archives of Allergy and Applied Immunology*, 30, 58.

Hughes, D., Caspary, E. A., and Field, E. J. (1968). *Lancet*, 2, 1205.

Knowles, M., Hughes, D., Caspary, E. A., and Field, E. J. (1968). *Lancet*, 2, 1207.

Levene, G. M., Turk, J. L., Wright, D. J. M., and Grimble, A. G. S. (1969). *Lancet*, 2, 246.

McFarlin, D. E., and Oppenheim, J. J. (1969). *Journal of Immunology*, 103, 1212.

Mackler, B. F. (1971). *Lancet*, 2, 297.

Paronetto, F., and Popper, H. (1970). *New England Journal of Medicine*, 283, 277.

van den Noort, S., and Stjernholm, R. L. (1971). *Neurology (Minneapolis)*, 21, 783.

Sensitization of Blood Lymphocytes to Possible Antigens in Neurological Disease

E. A. Caspary and E. J. Field

Introduction

Circulating antibodies to brain and encephalitogenic factor (EF) have been demonstrated not only in demyelinating disease but also in other conditions where there is reason to believe that destruction of central nervous tissue has taken place [FIELD, CASPARY and BALL, 1963]. The present work utilizes a newly developed method to demonstrate the presence of lymphocytes sensitized to particular antigens in multiple sclerosis (MS) and other neurological diseases as well as in normal subjects. Application of this same method to Graves' disease is described elsewhere [FIELD, CASPARY, HALL and CLARK, 1970].

Material and Methods

Blood lymphocytes. Lymphocytes were prepared from 20 ml samples of venous blood by defibrination with glass beads followed by removal of polymorphs with

174

saccharated iron as used by Hughes and Caspary [1970] in their modification of the method of Coulson and Chalmers [1964]. Generally there was a yield of about 10^6 lymphocytes/ml serum.

Guinea pig macrophages. A macrophage rich exudate was withdrawn from guinea pig peritoneal cavity by washing out with heparinized Hanks' solution (5 μ/ ml) 8–12 days after injection of 20 ml sterile liquid paraffin. The exudate was washed once in heparinized Hanks' solution, again in Hanks' without heparin (250 g for 10 min) and finally suspended in 10 ml of medium 199. The cells were counted and the volume adjusted to give 10^7 macrophages/ml for test purposes.

This macrophage suspension (containing 10–20 % of lymphocytes) was irradiated with 100 rad (Cobalt 60γ; at 56 cm from a 4,000 c source; dose rate 100r in 54 sec) in order to eliminate reactivity of contaminating lymphocytes [Field and Caspary, 1970]. Usually $80–200 \times 10^6$ macrophages were obtained from a 400–600 g guinea pig.

Antilymphocytic serum. Antilymphocytic serum was prepared in rabbits by intravenous injection at weekly intervals of suspensions of cervical lymph nodes of normal Hartley guinea pigs. This serum was the same as that previously shown to afford marked protection against the development of experimental allergic encephalitis following challenge with encephalitogenic mixture [Field, 1969], and to block antigen-lymphocyte interaction in a study of Graves' disease [Field *et al.*, 1970]. Agglutination titre of this serum was 1:1200.

Encephalitogenic factor (EF). Encephalitogenic factor used was prepared from fresh young human brain (subject blood group 0) by the method of Caspary [1963] and has the properties set out by Caspary and Field [1965]. Since it is a basic protein of histone like character, a histone derived from calf thymus (Sigma Chemicals) was also used as a control 'antigen'.

Basic protein from peripheral nerve (BP). Basic protein from human sciatic nerve was prepared in the same way as EF. It was weakly neuritogenic in guinea pigs when used in the same proportion of Freund's adjuvant as served to produce encephalitis with EF (though it is likely that manipulation of the Freund proportions and dosage of BP will produce a higher pathogenicity).

Electrophoretic measurements. Electrophoretic cell mobility was measured in a Zeiss cytopherometer. Observations were restricted to macrophages, readily recognizable by their size and liquid paraffin content under phase contrast illumination. The migration of ten cells was measured in both directions of the potential difference so that an estimate was made from twenty readings. The potential difference was 180 V and the current 7.5 mA. All measurements (to 0.1 sec) were made in medium 199, the temperature of the observation chamber being maintained at $23° C \pm 0.05° C$. Experience showed that different batches of medium 199 might alter the absolute migration time, though differences observed between control and experimental specimens were preserved. For this reason changes in migration time were expressed as a percentage of the control time, i. e. that of macrophages in the presence of the human blood cells under test without addition of antigen.

Clinical material. Measurements have been made on (a) seven patients in an acute episode of MS, (b) nine patients in chronic or ingravescent MS, (c) fifteen patients with other neurological diseases (GPI [2], Motor Neurone Disease [3],

Primary or Secondary brain tumour [5], Huntington's chorea [1], cerebral infarct with peripheral neuropathy [1], ? cortico-striatal atrophy [1], Guillain-Barré syndrome [2]), (d) thirteen normal subjects (mainly laboratory workers).

Procedure. To 10^7 macrophages in 1.0 ml medium 199, 0.5×10^6 lymphocytes from the subject under test were added together with a further 1.5 ml of medium 199 to make a total volume of 3.0 ml. 100 μg (in 0.1 ml saline) of antigen to be tested was then added, (EF, BP or calf thymus histone).The mixture was allowed to stand at room temperature (18°–20° C) for $1^1/_2$ h.

Where the action of ALS was tested, 0.05 ml was added to the 3.0 ml mixture of macrophages and lymphocytes and allowed to stand at room temperature for 30 min before antigen was added. Incubation was then continued for a further $1^1/_2$ h. ALS was thus tested in a dilution of 1 in 60. (Actually, as will be described elsewhere [FIELD and CASPARY, 1970] the method (considerably simplified) can be used to titrate ALS *in vitro*). As control, normal rabbit serum was substituted for ALS. In other control experiments antigen was added before ALS.

Immediately before introduction into the cytopherometer a specimen was shaken gently and examined for evidence of naked eye cell agglutination. Minor degrees were sometimes apparent after about 2 h at room temperature but did not influence results. Clumps were disregarded and measurements limited to free cells. Specimens were numbered and randomized so that the observer (EAC) had no knowledge of the specimen he was measuring. This also ensured that higher migration times (i. e. lower mobility) did not depend upon time lapse with opportunity for microagglutination.

Results

Normal subjects. Amongst normal subjects EF was found to produce an increased migration time in excess of 10 % in only one subject (GJ, F, aged 37) who later turned out to be suffering from Graves' disease. It is of interest that she, together with all those who showed an increase above 5 % (EAC, KC, DH, MK and EJF) had worked directly with brain material whilst the remainder did not. 10 % may be accepted as a generous upper limit for the normal subject, (table I).

With sciatic nerve BP no normal subject showed an increase above 5 %. Of the normal subjects, it is interesting that MK (3.7 %) had worked most consistently with BP during the last year. A few experiments with histone gave similar results.

MS patients (table II). All cases of MS showed increased response to EF apparently unrelated to clinical activity. BP on the other hand, did not give uniformly positive results, negatives being present in both active and inactive subjects. Three of the 13 cases examined for BP sensitivity showed a response lower than 5 % and a further 3 between 5 and

Table I. Electrophoretic response of normal lymphocytes
to nervous tissue and control antigens

| | Sex | Age | % Reduction | | | |
			EF	SNBP	PPD	Histone
JEN	M	22	3.3	2.1	–	–
ML	F	23	–0.6	–	20.7	–
KC	M	23	5.7	0.2	–	0.9
JP	M	23	0.9	–3.1	–	–
WK	F	23	0.6	–1.0	–	–
MK	M	25	7.2	3.7	–	3.9
MA	F	32	1.8	–	–	–
DH	M	33	8.5	0.8	–	–2.6
GJ	F	37	12.1	–	9.4	–
EAC	M	42	10.6	1.6	14.4	–
EF	F	53	1.1	2.6	–	–
EJF	M	54	5.3	–0.3	20.9	–
CB	F	63	1.0	–	–	–

EF = encephalitogenic factor.
SNBP = basic protein derived from human sciatic nerve.
PPD = purified protein derivative from M. Tuberculosis.
Histone = derived from calf thymus (Sigma Chemicals).

10 %. Over half showed a well marked increase (10 %) which was taken to indicate lymphocyte sensitization.

Sensitization to whole brain suspension was present in 5 of 6 MS patients examined. Unexpectedly one patient (DG, M, aged 21) showed well marked positive result with EF, but a negative result with whole brain.

Other neurological diseases (table III). All showed sensitization to EF and all except one (HU, F, aged 65) a positive result also with BP.

Antilymphocytic serum (table IV). When ALS was added to the guinea pig macrophage-human lymphocyte mixture before EF, the slowing which the latter normally produced was always abolished. When, however, EF antigen was added before the ALS had no effect. Normal rabbit serum was without effect in either case.

Discussion

The reduction of macrophage electrophoretic mobility in the presence of the sensitizing antigen [TURK and DIENGDOH, 1968] appears to have

177

Table II. Electrophoretic response of lymphocytes from patients suffering from multiple sclerosis to nervous tissue and control antigens

NAME	Sex	Age	EF	SNBP	Brain	PPD	Histone	
JPS	M	16	29.5	24.2	–	–	–	Acute transverse myelitis
GA	F	21	27.4	20.4	–	–	–	Acute
JEB	F	21	18.6	6.7	14.4	–	0.6	Acute
DG	M	21	20.0	1.7	1.9	–	2.0	Acute
BC	F	28	18.6	–	–	18.6	–	Acute
DH	F	35	18.8	11.0	–	–	–	Acute
WW*	M	49	16.4	21.8	17.4	11.4	1.4	Acute + peripheral neuropathy
NBM	F	35	18.0	3.5	–	–	1.8	Ingravescent
JLK	M	37	24.1	11.2	19.7	–	–	Chronic
JW	M	43	24.9	16.8	16.9	–	–	Chronic
SS	F	43	25.9	8.8	–	–	–	Chronic 3 / 12 after treatment with cyclophosphamide
EMG	F	44	14.7	0	–	–	–2.2	Chronic
AMcG	F	45	29.4	23.2	–	–	–	Chronic
MS	F	51	20.2	19.4	–	–	–	Chronic
NJF	F	52	24.3	12.1	–	–	–	Chronic
TMcK	M	53	24.2	8.9	20.5	–	–	Chronic
DC	F	62	22.7	24.0	–	–	–	Chronic

*This patient also had signs of a peripheral neuropathy.
EF = encephalitogenic factor.
SNBP = basic protein derived from human sciatic nerve.
PPD = purified protein derivative of M. Tuberculosis.
Histone = derived from calf thymus (Sigma Chemicals).

a mechanism similar to that operating in macrophage migration inhibition. Both systems require the presence of lymphocytes and the reaction can be abolished by inhibition of protein synthesis [DAVID, 1965; CASPARY, 1970].

Preliminary experiment showed that admixture of normal human lymphocytes with guinea pig peritoneal macrophage exudate led (not unexpectedly) to a slowing of migration of the macrophages – a form of 'mixed lymphocyte reaction'. Although differential centrifugation [KNOWLES and HUGHES, 1970] can remove these lymphocytes, it was

Table III. Electrophoretic response of lymphocytes from patients
with other neurological diseases to nervous tissue and control antigens

NAME	Sex	Age	EF	SNBP	PPD	Histone	Diagnosis
MB	F	42	21.8	21.0	25.2	–	Guillain-Barré
EC	M	48	20.1	24.5	25.7	0	Guillain-Barré
EI	F	48	31.3	14.1	–	–	Glioma
TP	M	49	21.7	24.1	22.4	–2.6	Sec. cerebr. tumour
JB	M	51	23.1	22.9	24.9	3.0	Motor neurone disease
MH	F	55	24.8	11.5	–	–	Huntington's chorea
AB	M	60	19.8	–	20.9	–	Brain tumour
TM	M	60	29.2	32.8	–	–	Periph. neuropathy and cerebral infarct
TC	M	62	22.7	16.2	24.5	–	Motor neurone disease
AW	F	63	18.4	14.1	–	–	Ca. body uterus
HU	F	65	19.1	5.5	25.8	–1.3	Cortico-striatal atrophy
JT	M	66	32.3	16.8	–	–	GPI
DN	F	69	17.7	20.0	–	–	Sec. tumour, primary bowel
JMcP	M	71	23.5	26.4	27.3	–	Motor neurone disease
LT	F	76	19.6	22.9	–	–	GPI (Chairbound)

EF = encephalitogenic factor.
SNBP = basic protein derived from human sciatic nerve.
PPD = purified protein derivative from M. Tuberculosis.
Histone = derived from calf thymus (Sigma Chemicals).

Table IV. The suppressive effect of antilymphocytic serum on the electrophoretic response
of lymphocytes to encephalitogenic factor

	Sex	Age		EF	ALS + EF	EF + ALS
JPS	M	16	Acute MS	29.5	0.7	31.0
NMB	F	35	Chronic MS	18.0	3.8	–
DH	F	35	Acute MS	18.8	0.4	16.6
JLK	M	37	Chronic MS	24.1	1.2	–
GJ	F	37	Control	9.1	1.8	–
AMcG	F	45	Chronic MS	29.8	2.5	–
MS	F	51	Chronic MS	20.2	0.7	20.5
				BP	ALS + BP	BP + ALS
AMcG	F	45	Chronic MS	23.2	3.2	19.3

EF = encephalitogenic factor.
ALS = antilymphocytic serum.

found simpler to expose the peritoneal exudate to 100 rad of irradiation which eliminated the reactivity of the guinea pig lymphocytes, without interfering with macrophage viability and this dose was adopted throughout [FIELD and CASPARY, 1970].

Antilymphocytic serum (ALS) is known to prevent the electrophoretic macrophage migration slowing induced by EF [FIELD et al., 1970; HUGHES, CASPARY and FIELD, 1970]. Experiments were accordingly set up to determine whether it might also interfere with the present reaction based on blood lymphocytes. Six experiments were carried out with lymphocytes from MS patients and from one control (table IV). Addition of ALS clearly restores mobility to that registered in the absence of antigen. If, however, EF was added first and ALS later, then the result was similar to that for EF alone. These findings parallel those of HUGHES et al. [1970] with sensitized guinea pig exudate and again suggest that ALS may act by 'blindfolding' the sensitized human lymphocytes [LEVEY and MEDAWAR, 1966]. They also support the view that what is being measured is a parameter of lymphocytic sensitization. It should be noted that throughout these experiments ALS prepared against *guinea pig* lymphocytes has been used and proved efficacious in blocking the reaction. There is in fact considerable species cross over in ALS prepared against human, guinea pig, mouse and rat lymphocytes [HUGHES et al., 1970].

Histone – a material with chemical properties similar to EF – never produced positive results. A few experiments conducted with a saline extract of human kidney likewise gave negative results.

The results suggest that lymphocytes which have become sensitized to EF are always present in the blood of patients with MS and other neurological disease in which there is appreciable destruction of nervous parenchyma. In 12 of the 15 MS cases examined, sensitization to BP was also present (taking 5 % as the upper limit of normal – table II). In the remaining 3 it is interesting that sensitization to EF occurred exclusively. Immunofluorescence studies have shown that rabbit antibody to human white matter attaches to both brain and peripheral nerve, whilst serum raised against peripheral nerve has much greater affinity for nerve than brain, but there is no absolute specificity [FIELD et al., 1963]. Divorce between the 2 (in the present 3 cases) suggest that sensitivity to BP is not simply because the latter shares antigen(s) with EF, but may act as a specific antigen in its own right. Since the majority of cases of MS show some evidence of sensitization to BP the question arises whether it results from a secondary degeneration of peripheral nerve or whether it is part of the primary disease. Whilst it is commonly believed that lesions do not occur in the peripheral nervous system in MS, there are in fact rare (and usually old) reports of 'degenerative' changes. No special study of the peripheral nervous system in MS appears to have been made though the literature is reviewed in detail by PETERS [1958]. Further examination of the peripheral nervous system with modern methods might be rewarding. A curious finding was that in DG, M, aged 21 years with acute MS. He showed well marked sensitization to EF but not to BP or whole brain suspension. This insensitivity to whole brain in the presence of specific sensitization to EF is receiving further study. Is is conceivable that this patient may have had a lesion involving white matter exclusively. Under these conditions sensitization to EF (known to be derived from white matter [LAATSCH, KIES, GORDON and ALVORD, 1962] might occur but not to nervous tissue as a whole.

Only one patient (HU, F, aged 65) amongst 'other neurological disease' failed to show sensitization to BP and all were sensitized to EF. There is thus no specificity with respect to MS but positive results occur as a consequence rather than a cause of disease. It may, however, be possible to reduce the sensitivity of the method so that only cases of MS produce a positive result in much the same way as the Kahn test is made to work as a useful test for syphilitic infection. Experiments have, for example, been made to determine the absolute number of blood lymphocytes required to produce a positive result and it may be that this may be less in MS than other conditions. Meanwhile, as is the case with circulating antibodies [FIELD et al., 1963] there is no specific association of EF sensitized lymphocytes and MS.

The method may be of value, too, in following the effects of attempted therapy in the disease. On one case treated with full doses of cyclophosphamide the remaining blood lymphocytes showed no sensitization to EF. Three months after the dis-continuance of therapy (and when the patient was much better clinically) sensitization had returned. Further studies with reduced drug dosage are proposed.

An interesting observation was made in 11 cases where sensitization to PPD as well as EF was looked for. Most cases showed sensitization to PPD though the prevalence of this is so great that it is impossible to assess the significance of the observation as it stands. There is evidence that EF shares antigen(s) with PPD [FIELD et al., 1963] and this is borne out by the finding in experimental guinea pigs inoculated with PPD that blood lymphocyte sensitization to EF occurs (unpublished).

However, this may not always be the case in man. One control (EFJ) with active glandular tubercle within the last decade had well marked sensitization to PPD but very slight to EF (and not to BP); another (EAC) who had been exposed to a case of active tuberculosis also had a high reactivity to PPD. However, both these subjects had also worked with human brain material. On the other hand ML (F, aged 23) had high PPD value (and she had been inoculated with BCG 4 years previously) but no EF reaction. In addition one observation has been made on a boy of 13 with a tuberculous pleural effusion. He showed a 21.7 % increase in migration time with PPD, 21.3 % with EF and only 8.5 % (i. e. just outside normal – table I) with BP.

The method used in the present work enables direct study of the sensitization shown by human lymphocytes using guinea pig macrophages as a 'marker'. It has obvious wide possibilities. Its application to the study of Graves' disease and the occurrence of LATS in both health and disease is reported elsewhere [FIELD et al., 1970]. In addition the method offers possibilities in measuring the effect of therapy in immunological disease, in titring ALS and in detecting sensitization in graft rejection.

Acknowledgements

Our thanks are due to Professor F. T. FARMER and Mr. M. DAY for irradiation facilities in the Department of Medical Physics in the Newcastle General Hospital; to Professor J. N. WALTON, Dr. D. A. SHAW and their colleagues in the Department of Neurology who gave us access to patients under their care; to Mr. KNOWLES and Mr. KEITH who took over the routine harvesting of peritoneal macrophages; and to Mr. D. HUGHES, B. Sc., who helped greatly in the production of the ALS.

References

CASPARY, E. A.: A fraction of high encephalitogenic activity isolated from human brain. Biochem. J. 87: 21P (1963).

CASPARY, E. A.: Unpublished observations.

CASPARY, E. A. and FIELD, E. J.: An encephalitogenic protein of human origin; some chemical and biological properties. Ann. N. Y. Acad. Sci. 122: 182 (1965).

COULSON, A. S. and CHALMERS, D. G.: Separation of viable lymphocytes from human blood. Lancet i: 468 (1964).

DAVID, J. R.: Suppression of delayed hypersensitivity in vitro by inhibition of protein synthesis. J. exp. Med. 122: 1125 (1965).

FIELD, E. J.: Antilymphocytic serum in experimental allergic encephalomyelitis. Brit. med. J. *3:* 758 (1969).

FIELD, E. J. and CASPARY, E. A.: J. Clin. Path. (in press).

FIELD, E. J.; HUGHES, D., and CASPARY, E. A.: Mode of action of antilymphocyte serum. Lancet *ii:* 964 (1970).

FIELD, E. J.; CASPARY, E. A., and BALL, E. J.: Some biological properties of a highly active encephalitogenic factor isolated from human brain. Lancet *i:* 11 (1963).

FIELD, E. J.; CASPARY, E. A.; HALL, R., and CLARK, F.: Circulating sensitized lymphocytes in Graves' disease: observations on its pathogenesis Lancet *i:* 1144 (1970).

FIELD, E. J.; RIDLEY, A. R., and CASPARY, E. A.: Specificity of human brain and nerve antibody as shown by immunofluorescence microscopy. Brit. J. exp. Path. *44:* 631 (1963).

HUGHES, D. and CASPARY, E. A.: Lymphocyte transformation in vitro measured by tritiated thymidine uptake. Int. Arch. Allergy *37:* 506 (1970).

HUGHES, D.; CASPARY, E. A., and FIELD, E. J.: On the mode of action of ALS; experiments on electrophoretic mobility of macrophages in experimental allergic encephalomyelitis. Clin. exp. Immunol. (in press).

HUGHES, D.; WOODRUFF, M. F. A., and FIELD, E. J.: Unpublished (1970).

KNOWLES, M. and HUGHES, D.: A technique for rapid isolation of macrophages from guinea pig peritoneal exudates. J. clin. Path. (in press).

LAATSCH, R. H.; KIES, M. W.; GORDON, S., and ALVORD, E. C.: The encephalomyelitic activity of myelin isolated by ultracentrifugation. J. exp. Med. *115: 777* (1962).

LEVEY, R. H. and MEDAWAR, P. B.: Some experiments on the action of antilymphoid antisera. Ann. N. Y. Acad. Sci. *129:* 164 (1966).

PETERS, G.: In LUBARSCH, HENKE, und RÖSSLE Handbuch der speziellen Pathologischen Anatomie und Histologie XIII/Z Bandteil A., p. 564 (Springer, Berlin 1958).

KEY-WORD TITLE INDEX

AUTHOR INDEX

Auth, Thomas L., 77
Arstila, A. U., 10, 26, 33

Beebe, Gilbert W., 77

Caspary, E. A., 140, 166, 174
Chambers, M. E., 140
Clausen, J., 38

Dean, Geoffrey, 76

Field, E. J., 166, 174
Fischer-Williams, Mariella, 112
Fog, T., 30
Frey, H. J., 33, 38

Goldberg, Irving D., 64
Hedberg, Helge, 159
Herman, Jean T., 145

Itabashi, Hideo H., 58

Kallen, Bengt, 155, 159
Kivalo, E., 10, 33
Kokmen, Emre, 58
Kolar, Oldrich J., 145
Kurihara, T., 26
Kurland, Leonard T., 64, 77
Kurtzke, John F., 64, 77, 88

Link, Hans, 121
Low, B., 159

Muller, Ragnar, 121

Nagler, Benedict, 77
Nefzger, M. Dean, 77
Nilson Olle, 155, 159

Palo, J., 10, 33
Parker, Julius A., 58
Pelliniemi, T. T., 26

Riekkinen, P. J., 10, 26, 33, 38
Rinne, Urpo K., 10, 26, 33, 38
Roberts, Ronald C., 112
Ross, Alexander T., 145

Savolainen, Heikki J., 10, 33
Simpson, John F., 58
Swank, Roy L., 43

Tourtellotte, Wallace W., 58